Bitch Goddess

The Spiritual Path of the Dominant Woman

Bitch Goddess

The Spiritual Path of the Dominant Woman

edited by Pat Califia
and Drew Campbell

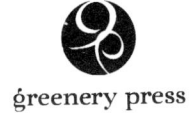

greenery press

Copyright 1997 by Pat Califia and Drew Campbell

All rights reserved. Except for brief passages quoted in newspaper, magazine, radio or television reviews, no part of this book may be reproduced in any form or by any means, electronic or mechanical, including photocopying or recording or by information storage or retrieval system, without permission in writing by the Publisher.

Cover photograph by Laura Johnston, San Francisco.

Cover and interior design by DesignTribe, San Francisco.

Interior photos and illustrations: p. 7, Kai Harper, San Francisco; p. 67, Lee Stranahan, Pasadena, CA; p. 115, Jimmy Malecki, Seattle; p. 143, Steven Fisher, Seattle; p. 183, Jack Cleveland, San Francisco.

Published in the United States by Greenery Press, 3739 Balboa Ave. #195, San Francisco, CA 94121.

E-mail: verdie@earthlink.net

http://www.bigrock.com/~greenery

ISBN 1-890159-04-2

Acknowledgments

We are indebted to many individuals for their support. Drew Campbell thanks Gina Gatta and the staff of the Damron Company, Janet Hardy of Greenery Press, J.J. Cooley, Scott Solik, Jennifer Williams, Devin Grayson, Brian Bouldrey, Ruth Marks, and especially Anne Bevilacqua. Special thanks from Pat Califia to John McClimans, Robin Sweeney, Ian Philips, Glenn Turner, the faerymen of Wolf Creek, and especially Val Langmuir. All errors or outrages are, of course, our own.

Dedication

This book is for Jennifer Williams, from Drew

and for Dragon, from Pat

Contents

Acknowledgments and Dedication iv
Pat Califia and Drew Campbell, "Epiphany: An Introduction" 1

Goddesses Ancient and Post-Modern
Lady Bachu, "A Dark New Bending" 9
Lori Selke, "Ruled by the Heart: Dominant Women, Strength, and the
    Tarot" 11
John McClimans, "Hekate and Me" 20
Joi Wolfwomyn, "Serving in My Mother's House" 23
Dossie Easton, "Kali Dasi" 30
Nicola Ginzler, "Mother/Mistress/Midwife" 32
Heather MacAllister, "A Bloody Muse: The Effect of Catholicism on SM
    Expression" 33
Ian Philips, "Sheldon Smalley Meets His Satan" 42
Jad Keres, "Song of the Heretic" 64

The Sacred Prostitute
Laurie Lovekraft, "Potato Peelings in the Shadow of Love" 69
Pat Califia, "The Dominant Woman as Priestess and Sacred Whore" . 71
Carol Queen, "Cleo DuBois Interview" 85
Maude Wolff, "Calibration" 97
MATAKLAR, "The Sacred Prostitute and the Three Kings: A Most Radical
    Faery Tale" 110

God/dess: Engendering the Divine
Bill Karpen, "Tellers of Fortune, Dealers of Fate: Dark Goddesses and
    Unmanly Men in Northern European Traditions" 117
Robin Sweeney, "My Life as a Consort" 127

Raven Kaldera, "Divine Intervention" 134
Dragon Xcalibur, "Goddess Be Care Full" 139

Bitch Ethics

Christina Abernathy, "Toward a Courtly Ethic of Dominance and
    Submission" 145
Liz Highleyman, "Playing with Paradox: The Ethics of Erotic Dominance
    and Submission" 153
Reilly, "Death as an Ally in Healing" 174

Rites of Passage

Lamar Van Dyke, "Becoming the Crone" 185
Lady Bachu, "Empty Me. Fill Me." 195
Catherine A. Liszt, "For B." 197
James Williams, "Goddess" 198
John Dabell, "Terror, Trance and Transformation" 217
Jezebel Strong, "Firewheel" 229
Sossity Oessa Chiricuzio, "Worshipping" 235

Contributors' Notes 239
Other Books from Greenery Press 246

Epiphany: An Introduction

Pat Califia and Drew Campbell

It is obvious that gender roles are shifting, partly under the pressure of feminism. But feminists differ on what aspects of gender roles or sexuality must change to guarantee freedom and equality for women. Feminist theorists have also been largely silent on the topic of what a post-feminist sexuality would look like for women. We take the position that as women become more powerful in public life, it becomes more possible for them to take charge of their sexuality. Rather than seeking equality by draining eroticism from gender roles and striving to make men and women androgynous by minimizing differences between them, we want to explore the possibilities a sexually dominant role has for women.

Feminist critics of pornography and the sex industry have frequently accused the dominatrix of being nothing more than a reflection of male desire and fantasy. This book is about women who see themselves as dominant because that is how they prefer to take their pleasure. *Bitch Goddess* explores the dialectic between the image of the dominatrix that can be found in the fetish porn produced for a male audience and the style, politics, needs, and conflicts of women who are trying to reclaim and create a new gender role for themselves.

Spirituality has been a strong theme in feminist theory since the inception of the women's movement. But discussions about feminist spirituality are often tinged with antisex ideology. Since a hostility to the body and the equation of pleasure with sin has been a major component of traditional religious thought, it seems strange to us that so many feminists have swallowed these assumptions whole without deconstruction. It seems obvious to us that religion has been an important part of a system that disenfranchises and shames women. We believe there must be a role for spirituality in women's lives, but this means we must discard some of the misogynist baggage of conservative Jewish, Christian, Buddhist, and Islamic teachings.

Bitch Goddess examines the dominatrix as a new icon of women's sexual agency and control. S/M challenges us to break through the spirit/body dualism of Western Christianity and other patriarchal religions and to reevaluate the body as the site of lived spirituality. The dominant woman overturns the stereotype of the domesticated female and the presumption of godhood as male. By presenting a variety of images of female dominance and divinity, this anthology explores the ethics and politics that our sexualities and spiritualities demand and celebrates the transformative power of the sacred in the sexual.

Just as the rowdy and joyous experience of liberatory female sexuality cannot fit within the walls of patriarchal churches or relationships, the ideas contained in *Bitch Goddess* could not be restricted to essays or articles. Our contributors employ many different genres to instigate new paradigms for women who are seeking power, pleasure, and transformation. Poetry changes as many lives as political theory or revolution. Sometimes the right sort of poetry *is* political theory and revolution.

Even the most firmly and aggressively patriarchal traditions cannot entirely banish the dominant feminine from their pantheons. From the resplendent Virgin, Queen of Heaven, who crushes the serpent of unbelief beneath her foot to the somber Mother Superior shepherding her novices, Roman Catholicism harbors enduring icons of female dominance. Tibetan Buddhism encourages devotees to meditate on fearsome goddesses and dakinis (female spirits) as well as their benevolent, nurturing counterparts, to integrate their aspects into themselves. Likewise, Hinduism offers Kali, the dark, consuming mother who dances on the inert body of her consort, Shiva, and banishes illusion and false ego. Islam offers us Fatima, the sister of the prophet Mohammed. Hasidic Judaism is infused with the sweetness of the Shekhinah, the bride of God, who goes into exile with her chosen people. From Judaism also comes Lilith, the first woman, who fled Eden and consorted with demons rather than submit to the boorish advances of Adam.

Goddess- and earth-centered spirituality has become as popular as it is controversial. Feminists have (re)discovered the pagan traditions of Europe and the Near East. In an age when the Institute for Creation Spirituality of Holy Names College in Oakland, California, counted Wiccan priestess and political activist Starhawk among its faculty, we can truly say that Wicca has come of age. Groups like the Radical Faeries and Black Leather Wings have merged pagan ritual and S/M sex.

Bitch Goddess is divided into five sections. In "Goddesses Ancient and Post-Modern," archetypal female deities such as Kali and Hecate, who represent the shadow, are examined alongside more accessible and nurturing images of divine and sexually powerful womanhood. This section features ancient as well as current and futuristic iconography. Of late, many pagan writers have been updating the tradition of holy harlotry, and in "The Sacred Prostitute," our contributors discuss the dominatrix and other variations on that theme. "God/dess: Engendering the Divine" contains explorations of women appropriating male personas as part of their spiritual path, the potential value of goddess imagery and folklore for gay men, and transgenderism as a goddess-based vocation. "Bitch Ethics" addresses the many moral conundrums that arise when power is exchanged, albeit consensually, in the sexual realm. And "Rites of Passage" celebrates the many life transitions which can be enhanced and celebrated in goddess-oriented, sadomasochistic rituals.

Unfortunately, there were many topics which we could not address here. We did not receive submissions which dealt directly with archetypes of dominant and sacred women in the history and current practice of Buddhism, Santeria and its related traditions, Islam, or Judaism. It is obvious that this topic is a rich and multifaceted one which deserves further exploration. Hopefully, Bitch Goddess will open the door for additional work about women, power, sexuality, and spirituality.

By bringing sexuality and spirituality together, we reach toward the source of our most primal human drives. Perhaps these drives spring from a common source: the hope of immortality.

Most ancient goddess myths center on the continuing cycle of change, the spiral of birth, growth, death, and rebirth that defines human existence. The goddess is the mistress of life in all its phases, constant only in her changing. Likewise, the goddess rules over our emotional lives with their waves of joy and grief, passion and despair.

In a well-crafted SM scene, the participants will travel this ancient road of change together, moving from fear and resistance to acceptance and exultation. Here the dominant woman embodies the goddess who controls our destiny.

Much modern-day pagan practice focuses on the goddess as Maiden – young and sexually ripe – or on the Mother aspect, the life-giving Creatrix. Very few practitioners have ventured into the realm of the Crone, the dark phase of the moon. Our deepest desires always evoke fear: our dearest dream is often a nightmare.

In SM, dominant women can reclaim this forbidden strength, guiding their partners through fear to rebirth. In the process, they themselves are changed, transformed by the awareness that death is not our enemy, but our strongest ally.

In these women, the ancient goddess is reborn, taking on new and surprising forms. Is she Hekate or Kali? The Virgin Mary or the Whore of Babylon? Does her strength come from the waning moon or the midday sun? There is only one answer to her, and that is Yes.

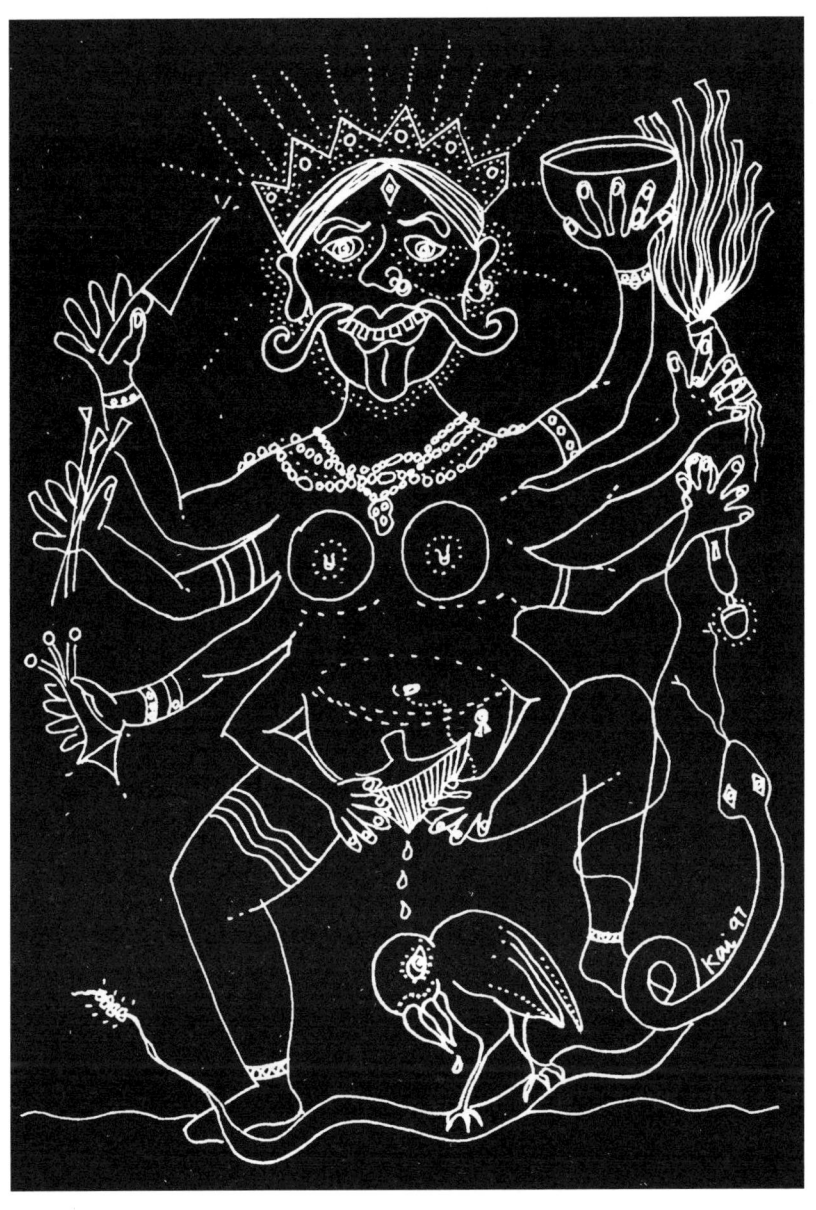

Goddesses
Ancient and
Post-Modern

A Dark New Bending

Lady Bachu

Step careful, new traveller!
Slip slowly knowing down,
into this well of shadowed faces.
Shed winter cowl and night hood and hard false will,
for here dive deep you in nakedness,
and dive again into surrender.

How wise, how foolish, to give yourself over willing!
A gift to me who hears the hungry whimpers,
cries urgent of a thousand souls begging to be taken.
To be swept by compelling hand without question,
without thought, without anarchy.

Test yet and test again and never win,
for it is not your secret wish that you do so.
Show me defiance bound, insolence begging;
And I'll provide the code of ultimate rebellion.

I will share with you a mutiny so profound,
it chills the soulless skin of politicians
and priests, and others who know it best;
They who perfect their abusive practice

over the clueless masses.
Hypocrites, they shake bony fingers at
its common guise, denouncing
those like me who practice
their secret shameful arts without deceit.

But you, you who called upon me,
submitted, ripe for the filling and the taking
and the stroking of soft furred places that have
never before known a touch quite like this.
Distended and exposed and peeled open,
swollen rich with long-held silent wants.
You will find your freedom here,
far from stranglehold of cotton and decision.

A question lingers with dominion:
How far to bend you?
Over bed? Over knee?
Over the steely discipline
of Your Lady who commands you
from the penumbra blueness
of your inner eye-lite self?

Bend to break? Bend to bend?
Bend to shape to a new knowing?

Ruled by the Heart – Dominant Women, Strength, and the Tarot

Lori Selke

The image presented by the Tarot Card Strength (number 8 or 11 in the Major Arcana) is most commonly that of a woman and a lion, standing together, her hands on his body, his mouth open, their eyes bound in a mutual gaze. This may be an unexpected representation of the concept of strength. The image itself seems straightforward enough, but it is difficult to see the kind of strength manifested in this interaction. This is perhaps because it is not an obvious kind of strength, physical and commanding, but rather more psychological, represented in relationship rather than force. This image, we will see, can have a deep resonance and meaning for dominant women, among others; it is a card of sexual power, and a card expressing a certain form of dominance. It also represents an often-overlooked archetype of female divinity and power, the Bright Goddess, counterpoint to her better-known sister, the Dark Goddess. These meanings are all intertwined, giving new insights into what it means to be a dominant woman.

Starting with the imagery itself, juxtaposed with the title of the card, brings up several useful questions to consider. What kind of strength does this image express? What kind of power?

The most common "summary meaning" of this card is that it represents inner rather than outer strength. This is often described as a more "feminine" way of wielding power, by enchanting or charming the beast, rather than the more overt, "masculine" expression of power. (Some versions of the Strength card show this more overt approach, featuring a man wrestling the same lion into submission.) Personally, I have some issues with the glib labeling of these modes of power expression as being "masculine" and "feminine." In her commentaries, Rachel Pollack offers a different way of looking at the division: "a different kind of power, not the ego's will, but the inner strength to confront oneself calmly and without fear."[1] In any case, it is an unexpected representation of power and strength to see a picture of a woman holding, perhaps even caressing, a lion. Nothing obviously prevents the lion, who is certainly physically stronger than the woman, from either escaping or attacking her. And yet, he (for the lion is maned and thus obviously at least nominally male) does not do so. The power here is implicit, not shown as fetters or force; it must be something inside the woman and the lion, something we cannot directly see.

Some versions of this card's imagery offer at least a hint of what this power might be. Bill Butler notes, in regards to the Brotherhood of the Adytum (BOTA) Tarot deck, "The flowers around her waist are connected with a garland round the neck of the lion thus implying some relationship other than domination pure and simple."[2] This is the first indication of the kind of meaning this card might have in regards to forms of consensual D/S relationships.

The sexual implications of this card's imagery and meaning are made clearer by examining some of the more esoteric aspects of the card and its symbology.

Traditionally, most commentators connect this card with the astrological sign of Leo, the Lion. Leos, born during the peak of summer, are (stereo)typically very stubborn, emotional, proud, and passionate people. The sign is said to rule over the heart, back, spinal column, circulatory system, and blood in general. The planet associated with the sign of Leo is the Sun, and thus the card symbolizes and expresses, in part, fire and solar energy.

The Sun is the center of our solar system, and the source of all life-giving energy for this planet. (Although it can also be very destructive, burning and blinding, too intense to behold directly.) In some aspects, then, the sign of Leo and the card of Strength represent and embody energy in all forms.

This includes sexual energy. Sex is one of the ways that creation and generation is facilitated (and remember that the Sun is the source of generative energy for this planet — just ask any plant); it is in and of itself a way both to gather and expend energy. In addition to this, and taking us back to the more symbological connotations of Leo and Strength, there is the importance of blood in expressions of sexuality; from first blush to the rapid heartbeat to the rush of blood to the groin.

One famous Tarot scholar, Aleister Crowley, has made the sexual connotations of this card explicit, by changing the name of this card from Strength to Lust. Many other scholars have made a similar connection with Sexual Magic and tantric practices implied by the imagery of this card.[3] The sexual overtones are those of active power, not dormant power; energy being used and enjoyed.

There is yet more to this image, however. As mentioned before, it invokes the archetypal figure of the Bright Goddess (as does the Empress card in the Tarot as well, incidentally. In fact, the female figure on the card Strength is, in several decks, dressed in an identical or similar fashion to the Empress figure, in order to make that connection more explicit).

A great deal of attention seems to be focused recently on the Dark Goddess and her manifestations, such as Kali, Persephone, Ereshkigal et al. This is all well and good, but it is not by any means the only powerful aspect of the Goddess.

Although the Dark Goddess still has her place in this discussion, she appears as the flip side or shadow of the Strength card. In her many manifestations She often represents undirected, "wild" power and energy. The image on the card Strength represents that same energy, except with direction and focus. Although the Bright and Dark Goddesses can be equally fierce, equally destructive, the Bright Goddess is energy with a vector, while the Dark Goddess represents that same energy without direction, focus, or control. The beast on the card, once tended to by the woman, is no weaker, but tame instead of wild, more directed, more focused.

Shekhinah Moutainwater describes this difference in another way. She sees two aspects to the Maiden. The Bright Maiden is the waxing crescent, she who is moving toward the Sun, the Amazon, the risk-taker, "the woman who dares." The Dark Maiden is the waning crescent, the enchantress, "She Who Pulls."[4]

Some examples of the Bright Goddess archetype include the sun-goddesses of various cultures, as well as a number of deities, mostly of Middle Eastern origin, who are associated in some way with lions, either riding them, otherwise accompanied by them, or, in some cases, part-lion themselves. Many of these goddesses are portrayed as both warlike, and involved with aspects of love and sexuality.[5]

The most significant of these goddesses, in this discussion, are the Babylonian goddess Ishtar and the Egyptian goddess Sekhmet, both of whom we will discuss further in a moment. Others of note here include the Greek nymph Cyrene, also possibly originally a Libyan goddess in her own right. (An ancient Libyan city was named in her honor.) The Greek sun god, Apollo, fell in love with her after watching her wrestle with a lion. Another Libyan/Egyptian goddess, Neith, is listed at least once as an alternate name for this card, in conjunction with an image of a woman wearing a lion mask breaking a pillar with her hands.[6] She is a virgin hunter and warrior, later identified by the Greeks with Athena. The Anatolian (ancient Turkish) and, later, Roman Great Mother, the goddess Cybele, is pictured in thousands of ancient artifacts sitting on a throne flanked by lions, or standing in a chariot drawn by lions. The Ugaritic/Canaanite goddess Anath, another virgin hunter/warrior, is renowned for her fierceness and savagery in battle, as well as for her love of it. Some of her battles are probably associated with fertility rites, and indeed she is described as grinding and sowing one of her opponents like grain.[7]

One common depiction of Ishtar shows her standing with one foot upon a lion. She was quite clearly the most important goddess figure in ancient Babylon and neighboring Akkad, recipient of countless titles and hymns of praise. One such hymn addresses her as "Shining light of heaven, light of the world, enlightener of all the places where men dwell."[8] Another describes her as "[She] Who dost make the green herb to spring up."[9] She clearly embodies both sensual and martial aspects; sometimes, these aspects are divided between her role as the morning and the evening star.[10]

Ishtar is also essentially the same figure as Revelation 17's great whore: "Then one of the seven angels who had the seven bowls came and said to me, 'Come, I will show you the judgment of the great harlot who is seated upon many waters, with whom the kings of the earth have committed fornication, and with the wine of whose fornication the dwellers on earth have become drunk.' And he carried me away in the Spirit into a wilderness, and I saw a woman sitting on a scarlet beast which was full of blasphemous names, and it had seven heads and ten horns. The woman was arrayed in purple and scarlet, and bedecked with gold and jewels and pearls, holding in her hand a golden cup full of abominations and the impurities of her fornication; and on her forehead was written a name of mystery: 'Babylon the great, mother of harlots and of earth's abominations'." Crowley specifically indicates that the woman in his card Lust, depicted as riding a seven-headed beast and seemingly in ecstatic abandon, is this Babylon.[11]

The Egyptian goddess Sekhmet is depicted as a lion-headed woman. Called "the eye of Ra," the sun god, Sekhmet represented the destructive side of the sun's energy, the terrible heat and burning of the desert sun. The most frequent myth told of her is of when she was asked by Ra to destroy his unruly creation, humankind. She proceeded to slay mercilessly and with vigor, for an entire day, and then revel in the blood of her victims that night. Ra later had a change of heart, but could not stop Sekhmet from continuing her assigned task until he had tricked her into drinking a large quantity of red beer disguised as blood, whereupon she fell into a drunken sleep and was unable to proceed further. This story clearly illustrates both the destructive potential of this Goddess, as well as the stubborn determination and single-mindedness associated with directed force and will.

The Bright Goddess archetype even appears in the versions of Strength which depict a male wrestler subduing a lion. The wrestler is usually identified as either Hercules or Samson. Hercules' name means "Glory of Hera," Hera being a Greek mother goddess who often oversaw the careers of various heroes. Samson's lion, after it dies, is discovered to be filled with bees and honey. Bees are another animal associated with the Sun, and summer; and the goddesses Cybele and Neith are both associated with the bee. The riddle Samson is presented with upon the death of the lion is also significant: "Out of the eater came something to eat/ out of the strong came something sweet" (Judges 14:14).

The Goddess underlying this card's imagery is the third strand of its meaning and significance. She is the one who provides direction to the energy, who brings out from the strong something sweet.

So, again, what kind of relationship/power is depicted by this card? It's cooperative – as noted earlier, the lion isn't restrained. It seems to be linked with sexual magic, in at least some forms and interpretations. It is based upon a Goddess who provides direction, guidance, vector. In other words, it's a consensual exchange of power, just as happens in D/S relationships, with the woman dominant, expressing the archetype of the Bright Goddess.

This is a cooperative, "consensual" power, not wrestling into the ground but taming, enticing; surrendered rather than compelled." This is a model for at least some forms of ongoing dominant/submissive relationships (although certainly not all). It represents a particular style of dominant/submissive interaction, between two powerful entities, cooperatively interacting in a dynamic of power exchange.

As a dominant, I want to provide the same kind of guidance toward personal growth that the Lady in Strength provides: gentle but stern. My own submissive has said, about this kind of relationship, "You are warm and bright; shine on me, nourish me, make me grow." And, at a different time, "I don't want this, but it's what I need." The Bright Goddess is not just an all-nurturing mother figure; we have already seen her, as Sekhmet, in the act of focused destruction. The lion has a certain amount of autonomy; it is free to move and act, for it is not restrained in a physical sense. It retains choice. But there is no question who has, and can use, the final authority and power.

The Strength card also represents an important developmental step in achieving self-acceptance as a dominant.

Many psychological interpretations describe this card as depicting the process of integrating the "dark side" of one's personality within oneself. This integrative process is very similar to the process many dominants describe as a key step in their coming-out and in reconciling and coming to terms with their dominant impulses. The card represents, in this view, coming to terms with one's own dominance and/or sadism, and being able to use them, and direct them, rather than fear them. The woman in the picture knows what she is, what she is doing, and what might result, and has come to terms with this; she has her own lion, within herself, her own fierce strength that she is now able to direct and use with awareness. She is self-assured because she is self-aware, and self-accepting. This is perhaps an essential step towards becoming a responsible and balanced practitioner of consensual dominance. Rachel Pollack says, "To release your deepest emotions with love and faith requires courage as well as strength."[12] For many dominants, sadists, and other SM tops, owning the desire to hurt or control another person can be very difficult. Expressing these "dark" desires is actively discouraged by the rest of society, and indeed are routinely labeled "bad" in one way or another: wicked, unethical, immoral, evil, or just plain undesirable and unattractive. Finding a route toward responsible, self-aware expressions of these "dark" desires can be a long one, and is a key element in coming out as a self-accepting SM top. Learning to express these desires in a loving and supportive way for all parties involved is part of the same challenge.

So, in the end, not only does the Strength card represent a model for dominant/submissive relationships, but it is a developmental model for dominants as well, representing the process of reconciling and integrating one's "darker passions" and giving them a place in one's personality and expression. This card combines the elements of sexual strength, ability to handle both one's own strength and that of one's submissive, and the archetype of the Bright Goddess, director and shaper. In this context, it is useful to consider Aleister Crowley's statement on his reasons for changing the name of the card from Strength to Lust: "Lust implies not only strength, but the joy of Strength exercised."[13] There can be few better descriptions of a happy dominant/submissive relationship, I think, than one in which both partners feel free to experience Crowley's lust, and the joy of Strength exercised.

> *Thanks to A. Martelli and S. Schwartz for their assistance both before and during the composition of this essay.*

1. *Rachel Pollack,* Seventy-Eight Degrees of Wisdom. Part 1: The Major Arcana. *San Francisco: Aquarian/Thorsons, 1980.*

2. *Bill Butler,* Dictionary of the Tarot. *New York: Schocken Books, 1975.*

3. *There is, for example, a strong connection between the identification of the Hebrew letter, Teth, "snake," with this card in Kabbalistic systems, and the Kundalini snake energy that is thought to be awakened by Tantric practice.*

4. *Shekhinah Mountainwater,* Ariadne's Thread. *Freedom, California: Crossing Press, 1991.*

5. *An excellent resource for further information about the Bright Goddess, specifically as manifested in sun goddesses, is the book* Eclipse of the Sun *by Janet McPrickard*

(Glastonbury, England: Gothic Images Publications, 1990). I found this book while this essay was in its final drafts. It should be noted that McPrickard has a rigorously anthropological bent to her work, and is rather dismissive of modern spiritual appropriations of the ancient myths she discusses. Nonetheless, this book is a fascinating and valuable survey of sun goddesses in myriad cultures and traditions, and includes an excellent discussion of why and how knowledge of sun goddesses has been suppressed.

6. Barbara Walker, The Secrets of the Tarot. *San Francisco: Harper Collins, 1984.*

7. *cited in Jessica Amanda Salmonson,* Dictionary of the Amazons. *New York: Paragon House, 1991.*

8. *Will and Ariel Durant,* Our Oriental Heritage. *New York: Simon and Shuster, 1935.*

9. *Assyrian and Babylonian Literature, cited in Barbara Walker,* The Woman's Encyclopedia of Myths and Secrets. *San Francisco: Harper and Row, 1983.*

10. It should be noted, as another intriguing connection to sexual magic, that Ishtar is one of several ancient goddesses known to sponsor sacred prostitution.

11. *Aleister Crowley,* The Book of Thoth. *York Beach, Maine: Samuel Weiser Inc., 1993.*

12. *Pollack,* Seventy-Eight Degrees of Wisdom. Part 1: The Major Arcana.

13. *Aleister Crowley,* The Book of Thoth.

Hekate and Me

John McClimans

Part I

In the Fall of 1973 I was invited to be part of a Dark of the Moon ritual in Lincoln Park, Chicago. Young and arrogant, I had taken to "working" with Hekate, despite warnings by several elders in the group I had moved from St. Louis to work with that I was too young and inexperienced. I ignored all of the warnings. I suspect that I didn't have any idea of who I was "working" – more honestly, "playing" with. In those days most traditional covens and working groups held Hekate in the same esteem that the Pagan community held SM spirituality in the eighties and early nineties. Phrases like "evil" and "sick shits" were common. I've always been drawn to the forbidden and dangerous. Being warned against Hekate was just the magnet I needed to be pulled closer.

The Dark of the Moon is the few hours when the Moon is not visible just before the first crescent of the New Moon. It is traditionally the time Hekate, Queen of the Witches and Mistress of Magic, is worshiped. Then and now, this is one of the most scary times of the month – for those who don't belong there.

I'm not sure I belonged there. I was scared juiceless. I wasn't going to be overcome by fear of... what?... a myth? I was going to prove that I was "man enough" to offer myself to this powerful goddess.

I remember standing in a circle with several others. The priestess cast the circle and invoked Hekate. It was cold and a light wind brought a mist across our circle from Lake Michigan, or perhaps from the underworld. I'm not sure how long we were there. I was shifting my weight from one foot to the other and wondering why I came out on a night like this. I was wondering when the priestess would open the circle and let us get out of the cold.

She was there! Right in front of me! If I had dared I could have reached out and touched her. This wasn't some "religious peak experience." This was Her, Hekate, and I had been strutting around earlier thinking about how I was "man enough" to... what? If I was ever to become any kind of a man it would be Her doing.

There are parts of this experience that I can't share with you. No, it's not secret. I just don't have the vocabulary to describe what happened. It wasn't a conversation. Hekate didn't stand there and make a flowing speech about what she wanted me to do. But when it was over, that is when I became aware of my surroundings again, I knew that I really had given myself up to Her. I knew that when I grew up, when I did what I had to do to become worthy of Her, She would allow me to be one of Her companions.

I came away from that Dark of the Moon and into the first light of a New Moon knowing that before I could worship this cthonic Crone I had to accept Her as Maiden and Mother. I needed to enjoy Her as a "young girl" and a "mature woman" before I would be able to enjoy her as a powerful Queen of the Witches.

Part II

For years I've paraphrased Lincoln with "everything I am or ever hope to be I owe to some woman somewhere." True enough, but each of these women can be seen as an aspect of Hekate. It would be equally true to say "everything I am or ever hope to be I owe to Hekate."

Throughout my life I have been "trained" or "civilized" by any number of women. I've eagerly sought the training. Sometimes begged for it. I've been rejected and accepted for more different reasons than I can remember. I've always felt the strong hand of Hekate guiding me to the women who I needed to learn from. I've been rewarded for following this path I accepted in Chicago with a remarkably varied group of friends and partners. I've been loved and I have been allowed to love more than I could have dreamed possible in 1973. In the company of these women I have come full circle. I've learned that becoming "man enough" was never my goal. I've been able to put aside much of that ego so I give myself to the "old woman" who is the young girl" who is the "mature woman".

> What will you offer her?
> Clean hands? A pure heart?
> Hers are not. She is not.
> She is an old woman.
> She has seen everything
> > done everything
> > endured everything
> She is responsible
> For everything.
>
> Then your least fear
> Is knowledge
> Of the whip by her hand.*

I am no longer scared juiceless. I have come to accept my role. Only Hekate could take it away from me. She won't, She's my main squeeze.

* *From "Winter" by Deborah Bender. It appears here with the poet's permission.*

Serving in My Mother's House

Joi Wolfwomyn

I am serving my mother. I am carrying her where I walk. I am carrying her into the realities of others, into where she wants to be.

I am serving my mother by being her horse, her mouth, her hands, her voice.

I am serving my mother when I sing, when I open the gates to her temple.

I am one of my mother's gatekeepers. I stand for her at the gate, I lift only the outermost veil so that others may enter into her strength and radiance.

When I am serving my mother, she cares for me and allows me to sit in her lap. Sometimes I am her channel. Sometimes I am her pet.

I manifest her energy, as presence.

It is a dance of chaos. I manifest her energy by bringing her dominance into presence, so that others may give her what they will, what she may want.

She is the terrifying mother. When I create terror in another, by psychic or physical means, I take them into her presence. I enable transformation, if that is what is chosen.

What happens in the temple is not of me. I open the gate, I guard, I wait outside, with comfort after the fear, after the power is revealed.

It is an odd dance of feelings, mother destroyer lover warrior.

My mother slays demons. I can only show her where they are.

I serve my mother by showing people their own demons, and leading them to her so they may make sacrifices of them.

Those who have had enough of demons will offer them to my mother. Some will choose to keep them. It is never forced. Those who keep their demons often turn away in rage. I wait by the temple gate.

Only sometimes my mother will catch me when I fall, but she will always hold me once I arise.

I have always served my mother. When I didn't know her, I served her. I was told it was wrong, that she didn't exist.

I was lied to.

My mother has many sisters. They all have servants.

Some of us serve at gates, some of us tend fires, some of us serve food. Some of us serve for lifetimes, some serve only for moments.

All service is rendered due. One cannot pretend to serve. If one claims a role, it will be played eventually. While I am bound by consent, she is not. She does not "demand" absolute submission, as that would imply there was choice in the matter.

One can choose to directly acknowledge her, but there is no choice in where you walk, and what her will is.

By serving my mother as gatekeeper, I have many aspects. There are no limits on how I play my part.

There are many doors, and no one uniform is required.

I am serving in my mother's house. My key opens many doors. Not all. Not even one in nine.

Sometimes the key is a word. Sometimes the key is a whip. Sometimes the key is a hand on the heart and a soft lap. Sometimes the key is a rattan cane singing in the air.

Sometimes the key is shiny and sharp.

Sometimes the door opened is not the one expected.

I am serving in my mother's house.

I am the machine and She is the operator. I am the house and She is the indweller. I am the chariot and She is the charioteer. I move as She moves me; I speak as She speaks through me.

The Gospel of Sri Ramakrishna

SERVING IN MY MOTHER'S HOUSE

The candles are lit. The altar is set in the west, a place of healing and cleansing. Set in concentric circles, the murtis (statues) are of the Hindu pantheon closing in, with Ma Kali at the center. All the devis, Durga, Saraswati, Laksmi, gather around her, with Shiva and Ganesha watching. Later, we will do this ritual, this puja offering for Shiva, and his murti will be at the center of the altar.

She who is the pujaree, the supplicant, the one who will pray and offer herself up to the Mother, is kneeling in front of the altar, chanting softly. On the altar in front of her, set in a semicircle in front of the murtis, are the tools we will use for her journey and transformation. The whips, and canes, and knives.

I stand over her, chanting with her, whip in hand. This whip I am holding is made from my hair, from when I shaved my dreadlocks off in sacrifice. We chant Ganesha together, invoking he who opens gateways and removes obstacles from the path. Our chanting grows louder as the candles and oil lamp burn higher, and the incense surrounds us.

I stand behind her, and gently brush the hair whip over her back. It is a beginning, a sweeping of her chakras, a reassuring softness that begins this harsh and beautiful journey. Tonight we will go through the number of whips on the altar, chanting Ma's name with each, until through this act, she as supplicant, and I as priest, reach a state of communion, and are at one with Ma and the universe.

In most SM iconography, the one holding the whip is the top. The dominant. I am a priest of the goddess in her aspect of the Dark Mother Kali, although Sekhmet has also been my guide and inspiration. I am her servant, and her submissive.

I was called to Ma Kali's service many years ago, when my brother and ritual partner, Kalyn, asked me to dance for her in a ritual of the yugas, which are the Hindu cycles of time. The world is currently living in the Kaliyuga, and will transform into the Yamayuga sometime in the next century.

When most non-Hindus hear the name of Kali, if they recognize her at all, it is with an image of blood and gore and demon-slaying. While She indeed has these aspects, She is also a benevolent mother, holding her hands out to her children in love and nurturing. Behind her nurturing, as a foundation of her kindness and love, is an implacability beyond most humans' ken. Hers is the immovable love of the universe.

When we began planning the yuga ritual, I had been pagan for many years at that point, and had been a pervert for less than one. In my years in the pagan community, I had done many rituals, both public and private, the way that all the books described them. I lit all the candles, sang all the neo-Celtic songs, raised the cones of power, and walked away from them wondering what I had done wrong. I found some level of peace and community, but no transcendence. None of the meditation techniques worked, and I struggled with that for a long time. I thought at the time there was something wrong with me, that I was doing something incorrectly.

When I first encountered pagan Goddesses, they were mostly presented as sweet nurturers, mothers who comforted and kissed away the hurt of the world. Mothers of solace, and little else. There are Goddesses like that, powerful and strong, caring and loving. They all have sides that are fierce, however, that are warriors and slayers of demons. No aspect is stronger than any other. All are her, her power and strength.

After I was asked to do this yuga ritual, I started studying Hindu tradition and culture. It is my belief that to work in a religion, one must have an understanding and respect for the culture it is in symbiosis with. I researched the shakta tradition, and found many mentions of rituals involving extreme sensory stimulation, and body modification. It was like a light going off all around me.

What experiences I had had with SM had been brief and unfocused. I felt like I needed to do this, but I wasn't sure why or how, as the leather scene I had access to at that point was limited, and very narrow in its range. Certainly no mention of anything like deity or spirituality were ever mentioned.

After reading about experiences such as the taipusam festivals, where people go through very extreme body piercings as prayers and offerings, and finding documentation of some of the sadhu ascetic practices, I realized that what I had been lacking in my ritual practice was a physical focus.

I was blessed at that point in my life by finding a circle of people who used SM as a ritual tool, and combined SM technique with trancework to achieve catharsis and transformation. I received an initiation in this practice from a powerful woman, Deon Giselle, who took me on one of the most profound ritual journeys of my life, and showed me the healing power available through a journey of the senses.

Now, years later, my room is my temple is my dungeon. In sacred space I help others find the divine within them, and offer all of my self and interactions to my mother deity. It took me a long time to reconcile, let alone blend, being a priest and a sadist. Mine is a goddess of paradox, of dichotomy. "Bondage and liberation are both of her making," said Sri Ramakrishna.

Mine is a mother of blood and light, birth and darkness, blissful fear and terrifying realizations. The smell and feel of change belong to her. She is that which encompasses all dualities, and in doing so, becomes more than any two things. It is only by knowing her that one can see beyond the duality of her universe.

As a priest it often looks and feels as if I am controlling her rituals. While leading chanting, whipping, or offering fire and blood, I guide the energy in the circle, however many people take part. All of my actions are in her service. I echo her in shaping power in ritual, be it a ritual of many worshipping, or a ritual of few in transformation.

The duality here is that while I am controlling the dynamics of the scene, of the ritual, I am in that same moment bowing my head to her will and desire; gathering the energy of my bottom, of the circle of people I hold sway; offering it up to her for her pleasure and consumption. I am not that power which effects the transformation, I am the horse which she rides upon, into the circle, into the body and soul of the pujaree. I am the one who holds open the gate to her presence, and not even I know what she will do when she shows her self.

She has given me the gift of the ability to open people to her presence, by song, by fire, by pain, and by sex. Every time I use the gifts she has given me, I praise her. I praise her not out of fear, although she is terrifying. I praise her out of love and gratitude, and sometimes I praise her out of anger. This sometimes strikes people as odd – to be angry at her, as if anger were not passion.

When someone comes to me seeking her, seeking communion through intensity, seeking to be pushed through pain to the point of illumination, then she has brought them to me to be their guide. By leading them, by being the dominant one, by being the biggest thing in their universe for a short time, I can take them to her temple door, and into her presence.

There are those who find her door, but do not enter. There are those who enter, and do not see. There are those who see and do not accept their vision. All of these are still her children. One cannot walk into her temple and walk out the same.

It is six years now that I walk her path. By books and temples have I found her, in unexpected places. Her lessons are rarely easy, her means often subtle.

I am finding my way through this, with my Mother to carry me.

Recommended Reading

Ajit Mookerjee, *Kali: The Feminine Force*, Thames and Hudson Limited, 1988.

Robert E. Svoboda, *Aghora*, Brotherhood of Life Inc. Publishing, 1986.

Robert E. Svoboda, *Aghora II: Kundalini*, Brotherhood of Life Inc. Publishing, 1993.

The Gospel of Sri Ramakrishna

The Chandi Path and *The Devi Gita*. Traditional Hindu scriptures. Check local temples.

Lex Hixon, *Mother of the Universe: Visions of the Goddess and Tantric Hymns of Enlightenment*, Quest Books/Theosophical Publishing House, 1994.

Ramprasand Sen, *Grace and Mercy in Her Wild Hair: Selected Poems to the Mother Goddess*, translated by Leonard Nathan and Clinton Seeley, Great Eastern Book Company, 1982.

Kali Dasi

Dossie Easton

Black skin, Scarlet tongue
Hard feet horny trample me
Beloved, Destroyer, my Mother
Your skin eats light
Utterly round Your hips
I sink in Your breasts, infinite softness
Hanging beneath the skulls of men
Your arms trap me implacable
In the language of crows You
Open me up You
Tear me down

Tigress sweaty over me, Your fur scours.
You turn me over, buffet me,
Spread my legs with Your great paws.
Your claws, sheathing and unsheathing,
Knead my flesh, spilling little streams.
Scarlet Your tongue, bright like persimmons
You lick salt in my wounds.

Your huge tongue
In the language of frogs
Rough like starfish

Licks my cunt, sucks me dry:
I am not ready.
I try to offer myself but You allow
No will, no reason:
I am not ready.
I am Yours because You take me.

Tails of snakes enfold me, muscles
Wrap my limbs, crush my chest, I cannot breathe
Your rattles in my ears are all the sound of the Universe,
        Deafening me.

Where Your rocks meet Your waters in thunder
Your cliffs are dangerous, my Lady
Your tides turn stones back and forth, clicking
Shaman's rattle, diamond back,
Demon Mother, Killing Moon
Eclipse me in Your infinite darkness.

With shining steel nails on fingers and toes
You lift me, shake me, split my skin
Spill my life in sticky red streams and then You
        Let go.
I land empty
Dry and rattling
I have forgotten that I am.
I must be
Yours.

Mother/Mistress/Midwife

Nicola Ginzler

Breathe,
she tells me, *Speaking as one who knows,* she tells me

Breathe,
If you breathe, you can feel it,

> she says, *Let the pain take you over,* she says, strong arms holding me close, my head buried in scarlet curls. My back ignites, bare flesh arching to meet leather. *Let the pain take you over,* she says, *Speaking as one who knows,* she says

Breathe,
If you breathe, you can feel it,
If you feel it, you can ride it,

> she whispers in my ear, *Let it take you over, let it flow into you and through you,* she whispers in my ear. *Ride it like a wave,* she whispers. I stand alone, the room is gone. I stand alone, waiting. Deciding whether I will step forward, ride the pain forward. *Ride it like a wave,* she whispers, *Speaking as one who knows,* she whispers

Breathe,
If you breathe, you can feel it,
If you feel it, you can ride it,
If you ride it, you can fly.

A Bloody Muse: The Effects of Catholicism on SM Expression

Heather MacAllister

Before launching into this treatise (of sorts), I feel it important to impress upon the reader that I am not a "practicing Catholic" in the doctrinal sense. My spiritual beliefs reflect many years of searching and are still growing and changing, as I hope they continue to do. I currently try to honor my ethnicity and my ancestors by research into pre-Christian Celtic and Mediterranean religions. On the other hand, I do participate in the Catholic rituals that I enjoy, such as Ash Wednesday and Midnight Mass on Christmas Eve. (This makes my grandmother happy, which is an added bonus). I also have a shrine to the Goddess/Virgin Mary as a spiritual and artistic work-in-progress in my home. Although my spiritual ethnic tradition may be Goddess-oriented, my cultural one is firmly rooted in Roman Catholicism. I used to feel guilty – surprise! – about only doing the "fun" rituals while not engaging in the everyday practices of a believing Catholic. Today, I think the church fathers should take a look around at their shrinking, unhappy congregations and wonder why so many of us only show up twice a year and at weddings and funerals. Vatican II[1] changed a lot of things; unfortunately, they removed the rituals that many of us found particularly meaningful (they've actually built Catholic churches without kneelers!) and retained the traditions that many Catholics, especially in the U.S., find offensive (such as the prohibition against birth control). Part of the reason this is happening is the phenomenal growth experienced by fundamentalist Protestant sects over recent years. In an attempt to duplicate some of that success, Catholic catechisms are becoming increasingly Bible-based and less ritualistic.

I have found the practice of sadomasochism[2] to be a surprisingly convenient site for the expression of my lifelong fascination with Catholic ritual. The rich history of the Roman Catholic Church, in its treatment of women, the body, and sexuality, leads very naturally to the disproportionate percentage of its members (current and former) within the ranks of SM practice. Although the teachings of the Church have changed a great deal in the last few years, many of us who grew up going to Catholic schools and/or in strict Catholic homes have a shared sense of the body and of sexuality as shameful. This is especially true for Catholic women. Our model of femininity is a virginal woman who gave birth through divine intervention. Catholic girls were constantly being told to hide their developing bodies and forced to follow ridiculous rules of (non) exposure in dress and behavior. A classic one (that I have recently been reclaiming) is the wearing of a Virgin Mary medal on the brassiere – the original intention being to dissuade any boy who had managed to get that far from his lustful pursuit. I find that rather than "protecting" young women from the influence of the devil, Catholic moral codes created an unbelievably potent desire for the forbidden that influences people all across the spectrum of sexual practice.

Instead of participating in normal adolescent activity, good Catholic children were exhorted to focus on how their sins added to Jesus' suffering. In contrast to the pure, spiritual ecstasy available from contemplation of the Virgin, we were presented with the beaten, bloody, and very carnal image of Jesus on the Cross. One of the distinguishing features of the Catholic churches in my youth was the huge looming Crucifix on the altar. The Protestants may have had large crosses on their altars as well, but they didn't include the *body* of Christ. Each week in church I would stare at the Stations of the Cross, fourteen[3] reminders of Jesus' path to Calvary. I wasn't torn between love of the pure and bloodless Mary and devotion to the carnal form of God in Christ. In fact, I have incorporated elements of both into my contemporary religious and psychosexual expression. Images of the cool, distant, beautiful Virgin adorn my shrine as well as the hallway to my bedroom/play space. In identifying with Mary, I am able to unselfconsciously express the maternal feelings I often deny in the rest of my life. I point out here that worship of the Virgin Mary developed among the Romans as well as the conquered peoples in accordance with certain local religious traditions (Artemis, the ever-virginal goddess, comes to mind). In Latin America (as well as in other regions) and among Latinos and others in the U.S., worship of the Blessed Mother has far surpassed that of either the Father or the Son. "Virgin goddess" does not refer to a woman who has never had sex; a more accurate reading would be a woman who is neither owned or taken by a man – an unmarried woman or a lesbian are examples. Additionally, when working as a professional dominatrix, I find the cold Ice Queen persona, the "frigid bitch" of vulgar description, very useful in my relationship with male clients, with whom I do not engage in sex. In fact, I prefer to remain fully, if sexually, clothed. In doing so I emphasize my divinity, my body as a temple, and his baseness, his weakness in the face of carnal desire.

Another way in which I affirm my body as the site for spiritual growth in a superficially Catholic context is with a ritual akin to the ball dance of certain Eastern cults/religions.[4] With the facilitation of Raelyn Gallina and the participation of a very dynamic group of women, I had the opportunity to participate in a modern version of the dance. After piercing the flesh and hanging fruit and bells from our torsos, arms, and backs, we danced to the beat of live drum music played by women musicians. Yes, it was painful, but ecstatically so. That very day I had ended my first love relationship, and I bled profusely where I was pierced over my heart. It had the feeling of one of the miracles that are sometimes recognized as such by the Catholic church – like visions of the Madonna and the little known but personally verified (by the author) miracle at the Greek Orthodox church in Tucson, Arizona (a bleeding picture of Christ on the Bible). None of my other piercings bled during the dance, but as I spiraled closer toward spiritual ecstasy, using my body, my flesh as a vehicle, the fruit that swung from breast to breast left a trail of blood in its wake.

I mentioned earlier the manner in which I delineated the boundary between a bottom's[5] carnality and my sacrality, as a woman and as a Mistress. The challenge for me is to enforce this dichotomy without adding to the layers of shame that certain aspects of our culture, both secular and religious, impose on all of us. I enjoy working with someone's guilt and shame, but I am also a firm believer in sexual liberation and, more importantly, positive body image. At the same time, shame and guilt are two of the most effective erotic tools at my disposal. I help my client use his physicality to express his emotions and spirituality. When I am working with an especially masochistic client, and I "take him down from the cross," beaten, bloody, and all too human, an intense spiritual transformation has taken place.

The dichotomy changes when I play with lovers. Although I occasionally take a male devotee/sex toy (I don't consider most [genetic] men my equals, so I don't use the term partner[6]), my primary focus sexually, spiritually, emotionally, and socially is on women (as well as female-to-male transsexual men). Although I still play out the Mistress/slave dyad, I am much more passionate in our power play. I allow myself to express my sexual arousal, and this persona is Bitch Goddess, as is my Ice Queen. I am often very mean to my sweet bottoms, and they love me for it. They, too, have shame and guilt and I am even more careful with them when it comes to healthy body image and celebrating their sexuality and carnality. Let me relate an entertaining story that I feel will illustrate the need for this sort of religiosexual play in the lesbian/bi women's community.

Visualize this: a hot summer night amidst thousands of queer women camped in pastoral fields in America's heartland. Some creative leatherwomen have constructed a mock Stations of the Cross. This party is organized primarily for curious women, women who are often fiercely interested in sadomasochistic play but are afraid – of the opinions of their friends, of us, of their own desires. Most of the attendees have participated in an "SM 101"-type workshop the week previous. Now it's Friday and time to put all that newly acquired knowledge to use! The Stations are staffed by carefully screened, experienced players willing to help novices along down the path of perdition. I had the honor of being asked to set up a station and together with the help of an unindicted co-conspirator we set up a confessional in the middle of the peaceful midwestern woods. I hadn't been planning on doing a station at all, especially one with so personal a meaning for me. In fact, I was traveling about the country at the time and had very little in the way of toys and props. However, with help from other Sationmasters and Sationmistresses we constructed a grotto amongst the pines complete with altar, a Bible (a Gideon's I happened to pick up in a hotel along my route), holy water, oil and ashes, and implements to drive out all sorts of demons.

Sister Sarah and I played a sort of "good nun-bad nun" game. We had managed to find clothing reasonably similar to many people's fantasy of a "sexy nun." Neither Sr. Sarah nor myself was quite ready for the response the Stations had engendered. The idea that one could "try out" different types of play was appealing to over 150 women that evening. As each woman approached our grotto, Sr. Sarah "lured" her in, using a sexy, sweet tone of voice to encourage her to confess her "sins." Many of the women were shy and needed to be coaxed. Several made up stories for the enjoyment of the audience. But the women I found most fascinating were the ones who apparently were truly confessing some deep, dark secrets. One woman told us, in a quiet voice, that she was having an affair with her lover's nineteen-year-old daughter. Another penitent admitted her erotic experience with her canine companion. There was definitely a difference in vocal qualities between the women who were sharing fantasies and those who seemed to actually be confessing. I firmly believe that these two women, in particular, were telling the truth about their lives. And where else would they go? Even if these were just fantasies, with whom could they share them?

It was after their confession that I, Sister Severe, would regale them with Bible verses and purge them of their sins. This consisted of whippings with varying degrees of harshness. Instead of "making the punishment fit the crime" as an actual confessor would, I tailored the penance to the tolerance level of the individual. Finally, I would anoint them with a cross of ashes on the forehead. This sort of gentle contact seemed to comfort the penitent after serving her penance. My partnership with Sr. Sarah worked well at this point, when she would encourage them to "go and sin some more!" It is my belief that each woman, even the ones who were truly confessing, left with the experience of telling her story without being judged, and perhaps experiencing an erotic thrill as well. In this scenario, Sr. Sarah served a more maternal role (Love Goddess) whereas I was the inaccessible, punishing one (Bitch Goddess).

I have recently had the opportunity to carry out this erotically charged drama on a more personal basis. The dyke in question was desirous of visiting our confessional but was "not allowed" by her lover to do so. Some time later she and I had the chance to play. I instructed her to confess all her sins of thought, word and deed. As she had recently split up with the aforementioned lover, she had some unpleasant things to say about her. I have found this reaction common among the recently parted. Be that as it may, I brook no such vilification of another femme in my presence, and let her know this in no uncertain terms. She naturally had other sins to confess, which she did eagerly. I instructed her on how to pray the "Hail Mary" and executed a thorough purging of her sins. By responding negatively to her criticisms of her former lover, I set a standard of behavior to which she can conform or not, fully aware of the consequences of her actions. She understands (as do all my bottoms) that I do not punish bad behavior – I ignore it. I don't need a reason to use corporal chastisement, so my bottoms don't usually act up simply in order to get my attention. In a scenario like the one I just described, several goals are achieved – the bonding to me of my bottom (a condition I find important in any ongoing SM relationship), establishing an enforceable guideline of acceptable behavior (at least within the context of the scene), and, of course, a fulfilling erotic experience for both parties.

The possible therapeutic role of power play in the life of its enthusiasts has become a topic of debate in the community. I have enumerated a variety of ways in which sadomasochism is, for me, a transformative experience. Perhaps you noticed that I utilize the concept of expressing one's needs that are not specifically sexual rather than saying someone is "working out" their problems. Although like all sex industry workers, my job has a counseling aspect to it, I don't claim to do therapy with my clients. The level at which most clients are relating to their sexuality is much removed from the intensity of emotion and spirituality I find with some of my personal play partners. First of all, I have to acknowledge the chasm of difference in the life experiences of men (clients) and women (lovers) as they relate to the body and sexuality. Secondly, the intimate and consistent nature of my relationship with lovers makes the chance that emotional and spiritual issues will arise in scene much more likely. Finally, and perhaps most importantly, my role as Domina/Mistress lends itself quite naturally to my being perceived as someone who can help my bottoms use power play as a metaphor – and the body as a site – for spiritual and emotional transformation. In addition, I have, at the instigation of a good friend, become a member of a "pervert family." We are organized in a surprisingly traditional nuclear family way. I act in the role of the mother, and the originator of our clan – who acts as father – and I have two "children," a boy and a girl (two of us are transgendered, all are genetically female). I hope to have a positive "femtoring"[7] influence. I leave myself open to constant revision of my boundaries and responsibilities, while at the same time honoring any contract I have entered into. In other words, I won't "leave someone hanging." Neither will I allow myself to be drained of energy that I need for my own development, spiritually and emotionally. I feel that just as a combination of factors, often religious ones, lead me to a dominant expression of god/desshood, a combination of factors in SM will lead myself and my submissives toward a spiritual goal. Something that I am discovering along my path is that the more I envision myself as goddess/domina/queen the more I am envisioned as such by others and the closer I come to achieving whatever divinity is available to us in this incarnation.

[1] *Vatican II was a meeting of Catholic clergy in 1969 that made significant changes in Catholic doctrine and practice.*

2   *I use the familiar term sadomasochism for a variety of reasons while acknowledging the observation of Rebecca Dawn Kaplan (as published in* The Second Coming*) that the term takes its name from the Marquis de Sade, an oft-romanticized rapist and wholesale brutalizer of women. Leopold von Sader-Masoch, from whom we derive the second half of the term, used a variety of inexcusable methods to force his wife to enact a "dominant" role with him. I am torn between "reclaiming" the word (or declaring it reclaimed based on its usage in popular women's language and writing) and substituting another term in its place. I have decided to take a third option: using the term (or its abbreviation) as well as using Kaplan's term* power play. *I believe there is room for both of these terms and more.*

3   *This, too, is in the process of being changed – the church is "removing" the station that includes Veronica, the woman on the road to Calvary who wiped Jesus' face with a wet cloth.*

4   *First of all, I felt it important to determine the occurrence of (or lack thereof) of such a ritual in European Christian tradition. I have serious questions (not judgments) about the integrity of performing religious ritual, including ritual body mortification, of a culture to which one does not have personal ties, especially without permission.*

5   *I use the term bottom where before slave would have sufficed. Although the image brought to the minds of many by the term slave more accurately describes my relationship with male clients and some female and FTM partners, it has in our culture taken on a racial and negative connotation. I model my Mistress/bottom relationship on older slavery models (including European and Egyptian), but until we live in a country where racism is a thing of the past, and adequate reparations have been made, I plan to use different appellations for those who serve me. Additionally, the term submissive is too specific and doesn't apply to all of my bottoms. As with the term sadomasochism, I encourage our community to play with the language so that everyone may feel included and no one marginalized. We write the rules here, let's make them rules we can all live by.*

6   *By this, I do not intend to imply that men should be subject to actual abuse or stripped of their basic human rights. I do not believe that men are inherently inferior to women; I am no biological determinist. However, the socialization of women and men in most cultures gives women the distinct advantage in compassion, clarity, utilization of intelligence, and other values that I consider crucial to human interaction. I make a distinction*

for transgendered/transsexual men, because most of them have been socialized as women and have been allowed to develop the aforementioned qualities unimpeded by masculinist expectations.

7   *As opposed to* mentor, *quoting Amiee Joy Ross (1992) (personal correspondence).*

Sheldon Smalley Meets His Satan

Ian Philips

Every time a world ends, the first and only warning comes in a dream. It would be no different tonight as the Rev. Sheldon Smalley lay down by beside the rivers of *Celestial Seasonings* Sleepytime® tea and dreamt.

*

He stood at the corner of Post and Montgomery, sometime in the night, maybe midnight, maybe 3:30 am. The battered grey blanket of fog had been pulled over the city once again. It bunched up in lumps in some parts; it was threadbare enough in others to see the stars beyond. Mercury lamps gave that comforting radioactive amber glow to every water droplet from the rivulet of piss flowing toward his shoe to the sky's underbelly overhead. Nothing unusual. He was downtown in the financial district. Except the streets were too still. Not even the telltale *pock pock, pock pock* of leather soled heels striking concrete. Not even the the distant clattering of a stray shopping cart. Not even the slow thudding heartbeat inside a signal box to announce the nearby traffic light would change.

Everyone must have fled. Those with homes to the suburbs. Those with apartments to anywhere they could afford. And those with nothing, to whatever doorways that remained unbarred. No, it was so still because everyone must be asleep. Except for maybe a few stray bands of office cleaners wandering on random floors in the random office buildings circling him. Nothing seemed unusual. Yet everything felt off. First, he'd never, before now, stood on the corner of Post and Montgomery in the middle of the night. He might have driven through this intersection or somewhere like it during the hours normal people went from here to there. To be honest, he'd have been driven rather than driven himself. He'd been driven most everywhere since his television ministry had been picked up by several cable markets. It didn't really matter. The point was that he wasn't the kind of man who stood on deserted streets some time in the night – long after he was sure he'd be asleep and long before he was sure he'd be awake. He had no idea what time it was. He only knew this was night. A foggy night.

Maybe there should have been some cars. That was it. It wasn't that he was the only living soul. No, there were no cars, not even parked. That was what was odd. No, it certainly wasn't that he was alone. He was surrounded by office buildings, stone and metal boxes and cartons. Nondescript but comforting. For each had a window here or there or maybe a whole floor lit up. He couldn't be alone. There had to be others. Go towards the light. But which one? There were hundreds of them. Which one was the right one? Where could he find help? But why did he need help? He didn't really feel in danger. A man who'd accepted Jesus Christ as his lord and personal saviour?! How could he! And this man, as unworthy a sinner as any other, had not only been saved but embraced. Given a special task even. And he shared this wonderful secret love with millions as he spread the good word every Sunday, at 6 a.m. on stations in Los Angeles and San Diego, at 7 a.m. on stations in Fresno, Sacramento, Stockton, Bakersfield, and Redding, and at 11 p.m. on two stations here in the Bay Area. And that was only California! He was his master's humble servant. He was the Rev. Sheldon Smalley. What on earth should he be afraid of!

He wouldn't have admitted it, not even here in what might have been his subconscious, that as his eyes widened and his upper lip and wrinkled brow began to sweat, he was slowly turning into one of the hellbound heathens he'd always chuckled at in those comic strips from Chic Publications. How he used to pass them out by the handful, before the Lord called him to labor in a larger vineyard – a televised one – hung with millions of souls ripe for the saving.

He was beginning to panic. Who was watching him? He was all alone. Or so he'd thought. Now that was all he hoped. But why? Which way should he go? Why did he need to move at all? He felt he'd be safest if he never moved – not even an inch – from where he stood. But he had to get away from the eyes. How many? Two, at least. Maybe more. A dozen. Maybe many more. Maybe every plate of glass in every building could see him. And behind each of these eyes were other eyes. Why was he so nervous about being seen? He'd been before the camera for years. Preached before thousands. Why now would he be afraid? Perhaps he'd buried years of stage fright, and tonight, here on this street corner he couldn't remember getting to, it had decided to surface. One enormous, *grand mal* panic attack no longer content to run silent, run deep.

No, it wasn't his imagination. These eyes were different from the millions before tonight. They weren't holding him with love, with respect, maybe, occasionally, even with awe and attraction. These eyes stared. Worse, they smirked. *Eyes that smirk will leer* he thought he remembered some great aunt whispering to him as a child. Yes, they were leering now. Then they laughed. A slow chuckle first. They knew a secret. A secret he should have known too, like his fly was undone. A secret that, if they'd liked him, even felt sorry for him, they'd have told. A common courtesy. But there was nothing kind about these chuckling eyes that now laughed louder until they screamed. He moved that inch. He didn't care about safety if it meant listening to howling eyes all around. Evil cartoon hyenas circling closer and closer.

Music. Beyond the eyes, he heard music. Faint thudding. As if a radio with some super bass thing were playing as loud as the driver could bear in his car, windows rolled up, passing several stories below a locked window to an apartment humming with air conditioning. It came from the corner across the street. The building stood alone from the others. In fact, it was a building while the others were boxes of steel, concrete, glass, stucco and sheetrock. It was not one shape, but a collection of angles and curves. Some of the stone was smooth and unblinking. Other bits curled into garlands or congealed into ancient masks for gods, for warriors, for even the occasional misplaced farm animal. Window arched beside window with an identical layer below and above. On the inside of this Roman aqueduct, curtains faded by a thousand suns gathered on each side of each window into the embrace of an emotionless winged brass cockroach. And both of these bugs looked up to the center of each arch where a small wolf's head blossomed – the lone bud left on a leafless trellis. All the windows, all the stonework pulled Sheldon towards the pillared portico. The garlands quickly grew thicker while the masked menagerie grew more menacing. Blank stares became scowls, maybe even sneers. The music too was changed. Less muffled. Thumping was no longer thumping. *Pa da pa dum. Pa da pa dum. Pa da pa dum, dum, dum, dum, dum.*

He went up the three steps through the center pillars. On the marble floor before the door was an oddly stretched circle. Even a simple geometer would have known it was an ellipse. Not Sheldon, however. He'd been forbidden to study much within the liberal arts. His parents had strongly taught him, hands on usually, that if it wasn't mentioned in the Bible, it not only wasn't worth learning, it just plain wasn't. Yet here an ellipse lay, smugly carved into the stone and inlaid with yet more burnished brass. And circling its outer rim like charms on a bracelet were figures and scribbles. And there were more scratches within the heart of the unacknowledged ellipse. To the simple geometer, these symbols were more arcane than most would like to admit. To Sheldon, they were undecipherable.

Once he'd passed over it, Sheldon pushed his way through the revolving glass-and-yet-more-brass door into the lobby of what must have been, by day, a bank. The ceiling had retreated even further away from him. Its squares honeycombed within squares within squares within circles within squares yet again. An educated liberal, or more likely a liberal education, would have whispered into his mind's ear – *early overblown Roman basilica*. But he stared at the ceiling unaware for neither had followed him past the door – the one unlikely to have this dream in the first place, the other unable to ignore the inscription in the ellipse.

The air, as still as stone, smelled of brash polish and cigarettes. The music had grown loud enough to make its presence known. It was all that moved other than perhaps his heart – no, too faint – the near-soundless snorts were coming from his almost-trembling nostrils.

Ooompa. Ooompa. Ooompa. Ooompa. The music had changed beat. It was quicker and closer. It came from the doors far across the white marble floor with the gold flecks that matched the white wood-and-gilt trim of the ceiling and the forest of hundreds of pillars and posts. The music sounded nice. Certainly nicer than the howling eyes outside. He wouldn't go back. So he walked forward. The *clack clop clack clop* of his dress shoes on the tiles was almost too loud. He tried to ignore the emptiness he felt all around him as he crossed what felt to be miles of marble.

The echoes reminded him that just that morning – was it really that long ago? – he'd clacked along with a crowd of journalists, lobbyists, politicians, well-wishers through the corridors of the state capitol in Sacramento. His idea – and he warmed just thinking this – *his* idea to turn the Defense of Marriage Act into a constitutional amendment had been hailed as an act of political genius by friend and foe alike. He'd learned the hard way not to quote chapter and verse from Deuteronomy or II Corinthians at every public forum. He'd learned to curb his usage of favorite phrases like "Adam and Eve, not Adam and Steve," "abomination," "pedophile," "child molester," "culture war," "Satanic lesbian witches," "mental illness," "God's divine retribution." Sure they'd been crowd-pleasers. But he was out to wow a much larger crowd now. Of course, he wanted to stop the radical homosexual agenda dead in its tracks. Who didn't? But there was something greater behind his "Endangered American Families Amendment." It was time that Christian soldiers all across this great land knew there were other generals in God's army besides that cherub Ralph Reed. And they *had* begun to take notice. Why just today he'd had breakfast with the Governor and lunch with the Assembly

Speaker. It was only a matter of months before he'd be praying with the President in the Oval Office. Yes, he was going to make it to the mountaintop this time.

After hours, days, a million *ooompa*s, he made it to the other side. The white-washed and gilded doors reached up to be closer to the still-retreating ceiling. He turned the knob and pushed one of the doors back. The room beyond was as dim as the room he stood in was bright. The air smelled even more of cigarettes. All he could make out was a vast desk that like everything around him had white wood and gold trim. He closed the door. When he did, the music stopped. He was startled at the stillness. Except for the ugly desk, the enormous room was empty. He began to walk towards it when he heard a click.

He turned as he heard the door open behind him. He wasn't alone. He'd been right about the eyes. That was the last thing he remembered believing clearly. For when his own eyes took in the person in the doorway, time and synapses and whatever else that usually ran smoothly derailed. Seconds and thoughts began to tumble from the track one by one. It was just like any other accident. The event happened in an instant; the effects would play themselves out forever.

He stood looking down on an old Mexican cowboy. Maybe he wasn't Mexican. He looked Mexican. For Reverend Smalley, this was anyone with brown skin and black hair living south of Texas – all the way to the tip of Patagonia. In fact, his only attempts to acknowledge any Latino presence in San Francisco had been to avoid the Mission district, day or night, to fight Army Street's renaming to César Chavez, and to ignore his wife while she watched that Linda Ronstadt special on the local PBS station.

Despite this doubt, he was certain, very certain, even in such dim light, that the man was very old and very little. Old was an epithet he was becoming used to, but little he'd understood all his life. Sheldon was no more than five feet three inches himself, except in the eye of the television camera. But now he no longer felt alone or small. In fact, this new arrival made him feel physically, morally and racially superior. The man pushed the large black leather sombrero back off his head until its stringy little arms clung around his neck. As Sheldon's eyes focused, his thoughts began to blur even faster. This he might be a she.

The face was both childlike and ancient, an odd combination he'd seen before in the features of the newborn and the nearly dead. Forehead and chin were broad and round while the cheek bones and nose were sharp and narrow. The skin thickened and cracked with wrinkles around the eyes and mouth, but it ran as thin and smooth as an onion's over the cheeks and forehead. It was not one color, not one shade, more a desert ridge of layered reds, oranges, grays, blacks, blues beneath a surface of sun-stained brownness.

If it was a he, then he had the faintest black moustache and a few whiskers on his chin. But these slight hints of masculinity combined with the jet black eyeshadow and mascara convinced Sheldon this he must be a she – or worse – a pathetic female impersonator.

He could observe her face so well because her hair had been pulled tightly behind her head into a bun, a miniature version of the sombrero now sleeping on her back. It was dyed. Black. *No*, he thought, *darker even*. As dark as when one walked, as he once had, out of a too-brightly lit cabin into the forest. Alone in the too-dark-darkness, too blinded to see any other shapes. Only sense their presence. Feel their shadows. Smell their closeness. Her whole small body was covered in leather dyed that same shade of too-black black. If pressed to describe her style of dress, he would have had even more difficulty than he'd had with naming geometrical shapes. To Sheldon, she simply looked like a member of a malevolent mariachi band or a motorcycle gang.

As his eyes had eventually adjusted to the dark outside the cabin so he could see the millions of stars in that night's sky, so now he began to notice little grinning silver skulls buttoning every hole and studding every seam of her leathers. He stopped. He could only stare. A large silver phallus, a gargantuan *milagro*, pointed out from her – *please, let it be a her* – crotch.

He trembled. He was confused. *What is it? What does it want with me?*

Her bony hands moved. They were speckled with liver spots and silver rings. They reached for the phallus. Sheldon's eyes had never moved from it. Suddenly all he could see were the blue threads of her veins, barely hidden beneath the skin. He couldn't tell if she'd unscrewed the phallus or unbuttoned it or slipped it off like a garter. All he understood was that it was glinting in her hands and then he heard it thunk hard on the edge of the desk. She turned towards him again. He realized her pants were not pants but chaps like a cowboy's. And beneath them was only her well-worn flesh. Where the lone silver bullet had stood there was only a tuft of pubic hair the color of steel wool. *How disgusting, that whore is flashing me,* he thought.

He was shocked. Here he was, the Reverend Sheldon Smalley, trapped in a room with some perverted old Mexican hag. He tried dismissing her from his thoughts with every name he could curse her with, and he knew many from his childhood in Fresno. But none had any effect on her presence. She was different. She was not of this world. She was an affront to the laws of nature. God's very laws! Such an abomination in the sight of the Lord could only be a demon, a servant of Satan. Now, Sheldon was angry. Why hadn't Satan come himself? Instead, he'd sent this old maid to terrify him.

Satan, just the thought of him, puffed Sheldon up with the confidence he needed to confront whatever this thing was. He would use His words to drive out this spirit. "Devil," he bellowed in his Sunday best, "thy name is legion, and, in the name of our Lord, Jesus Christ, I cast you out."

"Nice try, padre," she smiled as she looked directly into his eyes. "But I'd save that exorcism for the next available herd of swine. I'm fresh out since I scared away today's delegation of California Republicans. Forgive the form, it wasn't intended for you. But it always scares *la mierde* out of Governor Wilson."

Sheldon paled.

"Oh, I'm so sorry, my little one. Petie's session ran over and I had no time to change." She stopped now that she reached the opposite side of the vast desk. She turned towards him, lowered her eyes and her presence. They both stood downcast. "Perhaps, I could fold some laundry – yes? – make breakfast for your children – yes? – or I could just sit silently slapping out tortillas – yes? Would you like that, *don Sheldon?*"

She opened a humidor that had sprung fully formed from the field of green leather on the desktop. She took out a cigar as fat as a baby's thigh. She held it out towards him. He shook his head and his backcombed hair, a white shell covering his pink skin, wobbled to decline the offer as well. She lit up and pulled in several drags.

"Care for some scotch. No? How about some blood of Christ. Oh, how catholic of me! Forgive me." She whispered to her fist, now parallel to her face. Her thumb, jutting out from it as a bony lower lip, moved. "*Ego te absolvo.*" She looked up at Sheldon and smiled. "Let me guess, you'd prefer some grape juice in a paper shot glass."

He tried to scowl through her as she puffed away.

"Don't judge me, Reverend. No one I cared for was exploited in the creation of this masterpiece." She rolled the cigar between her thumb and forefinger as she exhaled. "I have a little plantation not far from here where little fair-skinned old men, just like you, shrivel up in the sun almost as fast the tobacco leaves." She offered it towards him once again.

He said nothing.

She began the long walk around the desk back to him, a demonic Rudolph, the cigar's burning tip lighting her way.

"So, *que paso*, Smalley." She ran her hands along the lapels of his gray polyester suit while she whispered, "My, my, my. The latest in urban puritan. Don't you look dour. Just come from a witch burning?" She jerked him down towards her teeth and spit out, "You know you've been fucking with the wrong side, don't you?" She let go.

"Ah, but that's why you're here isn't it." She wiped her palms along her thighs, then shook to get whatever still stained them off. "First things first. We'll get to the fun stuff later. Would you be more comfortable if I changed into something less comfortable for me? I could take the shape of Carrie Nation. Now, while I must agree with you, Shelly, that an axe *is* an amazing fashion accessory," she paused. "You – no, I guessed right – you have no idea who she is. Cotton Mather? John Calvin? Zwingli's definitely out then. How about good old *Miss Diet of Worms of 1521*, little Marty Luther." Her leathers cracked and popped as she clasped her hands together. "Oh, my god, here I stand..." she pleaded heavenward with the subtlety of a silent movie star. "I can do no more. Poor little old me, just 95 theses and a prince's army, ready to kick the holy fuckin' ghost out of anyone who disagrees with me." She turned her glance Sheldonward. But her black eyes met only the stern stare of his blank, bloodshot, blue eyes. "Isn't there any other disgruntled Protestant zealot you'd recognize besides yourself?"

"No words when the camera sleeps, o holy one. Well, then I'll just keep this form. It suits my mood." She jumped onto the side of her desk with a *thwack* as the leather of her pants greeted its kin stretched across her desk. "Welcome to your nightmare, *señor* Smalley. Would you like it hot or mild? For here or to go?" She laughed softly so that only the sides of her darkened lips, the color of wet clay, slipped upwards.

"I know. You can't take your eyes off me. You never thought someone non-white and over 25 could look so hot in leather. Surprise! And there are many other things of which you've never been aware that you will be soon. Of course, *mi hija*, if you listen to your spider grandma, they'll only hurt in all the right ways in all the right places."

She locked eyes with him, then looked down into her lap knowing his gaze would follow hers. She spread her legs even wider as she slowly slid back another inch from the edge of the desk. "It's a dick. You want to hold it? Go ahead, touch it." She crooked her right index finger under it, raising its head, then she straightened her finger and it flopped back into its nest of hair. "It won't bite. I will. It won't. You look confused, dear. We've been talking about dicks, Rev. Smalley. Mine, not yours. Or do you prefer the more clinical penis – yes, yes – how insensitive – this clinical penis doesn't bite. No teeth. See. Nor my vagina. Disappointed, eh, *mi hija*? Perhaps since *abuelita* is so old, all the teeth have fallen out. I can read the headlines now – *Travesty or Tragedy in the Underworld: Rev. Sheldon Smalley gummed to death by a vagina-no-longer-dentata.* Story at eleven." She held her cigar like a microphone and spoke into the smoking end. "Then at last, then at last, thank god almighty, then at last, my Smalley, you'd finally get a teensy-weensy taste of the fame you've mistaken for heaven."

He emitted a harumpf that sounded very little like a harumpf and very much like a heavy fart muffled by a thick mattress or a cushion in a chair. *She is not Satan,* Sheldon thought. *I will sit here until he arrives. Sending some minor demon, really. Lord, strengthen me to endure this trial. With your angels watching over me, Father, I will not break. I will not falter. I will not betray you. Sinner that I was and always have been, Lord, I'm yours now. Tell me how I can serve you here.*

"Disgusting." She put out the cigar in her palm with one swift twist. "You think your god's going to come rushing over for that half-assed attempt at prayer. Smelly Shelly, honey, you make one pathetic bottom. Throw you whole soul into it. Burn with praise or fear or desire." She pointed the blackened end of the cigar at him. "No, no, *mi hija*, I didn't say burn those you fear or desire. Burn *with*. *With*, dear." She finally laid the cigar to rest in a brass ashtray that had sprouted from the desktop as magically as the humidor.

"Reverend Smalley, you may find this an odd question, considering your profession and all, but do you know what an angel is? Right, right, a white person with wings." She slapped both her palms flat on the desk. The sound echoed. "Wrong. A being so awake to the desire to create that it burns. You could become an angel, still, instead of what you're settling for. Think about it. You could be your very own burning bush." She let both her hands slide well behind her and she leaned back on her arms. "I'm no shrink, Rev., but I'd say it's time to turn off that old projector of yours. Otherwise someone might kill you before you kill them."

He squeezed this idea into a little gun metal gray box and then stuffed that between the oatmeal gray layers of what a coroner would later claim was a brain.

"I felt that," smiled Sheldon Smalley's satan. "Daddy's little girl was listening."

There she goes again, that old wetback cunt, calling me girl. "Get thee behind me...."

"Oh, here we go again. All those lines from the Mount of Temptation story you've waited your whole pastoral life to use against the devil." She swallowed a yawn. "But answer me this. What could I offer you that you haven't already sought and taken? Power over the kingdoms of earth? Wealth? Fear? Death to your enemies? You have no need of a satan. You're the one who's everywhere. Your armies, the herds of the righteous, are legion. Me?" She lightly kicked the desk with the backs of her boots. "I'm here alone. Able only to inflict a little pain, a little remorse, a little poetic justice long after the deeds are done. Where's the terror in that?"

They sat silently staring at each other while her kicks kept track of the passing minutes.

"Why am I here?" he said as his whole body finally blinked. She stopped kicking.

"It was time one of us had a talking with you, and I manifested the short end of the stick."

He asked again. "Why am I here?"

"You've been here before, many times."

"No, I haven't. I've never stepped inside this bank before."

"Bank? You think you're in a bank?" she looked puzzled at the simplicity of his statement. Then she glanced around the underworld and laughed. "Ah, yes, the decor. Welcome to First Infernal. Will you be opening or closing your account today?" She laughed softly, encouragingly, hoping Sheldon was just playing dumb. He remained silent. Her face slowly hardened into a mask of pity. "You really have no idea where you are." A chair of white wood and gilt trim with a green leather seat and back now crouched beside him. Sheldon sat.

"Hell."

"Hell? This is your heaven. Surprise number two! All those years of wasted torment and tribulation, finding and seeking. I've found your kind bore easily of open desires. You've never enjoyed any pleasures on earth unless you stole them when you thought I wasn't looking. So I redecorated. I bulldozed the garden of earthly delights and buried everything under a hearty schmear of concrete. Haven't had a complaint yet."

"Why would I want my heaven to be a bank?"

"Don't ask me. You're the Protestant."

"If this is heaven, where's Jesus?"

"Like he'd want to hang out with a bunch of uptight assholes in a bank."

"I sympathize with you, demon. You will never look upon the glorious face of the Lamb of God."

"What makes you think you're not looking at that very face right now?"

"You sicken me."

"Me? You're the little infectious disease. Not me!"

"Tell Lucifer I will speak only to him."

"Oh, and all I get out of you is your name, rank and favorite serial killer?"

"I will only speak with Satan."

"Not in."

"Where is your master?"

"I am my lord and master."

"What is your name?"

"Why? Do you want to report me to my supervisor?"

"What is your name, bitch?"

"That's definitely one of my favorites. I have as many others as I have forms."

"Like Beelzebub. Mammon. Satan."

"No, no, no! What is your obsession with Satan, padre? You always want to talk with 'The Man,' don't you? Even when it's obvious the man's been gone for several spins of the cosmic wheel. Still you and so many others keep feeding that concept with your energy. I myself have no idea how I first, if you believe in such things as first, got here. All I'm certain of is that each year I grow a little stronger. Thanks to all those prayers, fears, hopes from all those people taught by you and your kind that they are no more than powerless pawns in a devil/god champion chess match. They hand it over to me, and I hate to see energy lie around idly – puritan energy will do that to you. So here I am – buffer, butch and bent on giving my children a good time."

"You mean you're in charge?"

"I'm, more or less, the zoo keeper."

"So you are Satan! Or the son of Satan or daughter or something!"

"When are you going to get it?! This isn't hell. I'm not Satan. I'm just the embodiment of your unwanted fears and passions."

Sheldon recited the twenty-third psalm.

"Great. Yet another love letter to god. Of course, it doesn't really matter. It's all falling on deaf ears." She smiled as if remembering a private joke between herself and a lover. "Deaf ears. You humans, I swear you'll personify anything, even the void."

"God knows all, sees all, hears all."

"Then he has an awful response time. Worse than 911 in a 'bad neighborhood.' When, old man, was the last time you remember him doing a walk-on? And I know why. Aren't you the least bit curious?"

Sheldon sat unmoved.

"Nice imitation of a stone tablet. C'mon, Friar Tuck, don't you want to know. I know something you don't know. I know something you don't know." She had begun to kick the desk again. "Ah, the silent treatment only works if I couldn't read your every thought. And since most of your thoughts are someone else's and since we've had this conversation a million times in a million different forms, I'll forgive myself for cutting to the chase and telling you all the answers." She stopped kicking to preface what she was about to say.

"This ain't hell. I'm not Satan. He hasn't been in since four – no, I think it was five, yes, five – worlds ago."

Thus spake the devil to the tele-evangelist, "God and Satan, dear boy – dear little malignantly mutated egg of your mother – they were lovers the whole time. All of this," she threw her small arms out wide until her leather jacket creaked, "was to get the other's attention, stir the other's passion, a game, a way to pass that which for them never passes. But they grew bored and left this universe so many longs ago for another. Why not? This play has happened so many times. And it will over and over again. So now there are no headliners hanging around. Does it matter? Sometimes some blob gets to your level, sometimes it evolves well past you. But you and I always end up having the same conversation about the same topic: good and evil. It never gets scripted differently. No matter the matter, I always get caught up in some version of this passion play for particles."

She paused and noticed him. He looked bored. Actually, his small blue eyes, small even behind his thick glasses, looked disconnected from his brain. They didn't roll or shake. They didn't twitch. They didn't do anything.

"C'mon Shelly. Don't blank out on me, *mi hija*. Right, right, take me to your leader – the one hung with a Y chromosone. Okay. I'd hoped to avoid that. Walk with me, my teensy weensy tiny whiny one. Your spider grandma is taking you to a fiesta!"

Anything would be better than this, he thought sleepily. He followed the black leather dot as she bounced down a long, even darker hall. The music had begun again. *Ticky ticky ticky ticky ticky ticky, ticky tat, ticky tat*. He could hear trumpets and laughter. They stood before doors even wider and taller and whiter than before. He guessed from the noise, hoped, there must be hundreds of people on the other side.

"Before we go in and party down, let's finish the talk we've both come here to have. It's fine by me if you don't say anything. I'm beginning to enjoy having all this air time to myself. Amazing, isn't it? I once was blind but now I see why you've always avoided any televised debates. So wise for one so stupid, my Sheldunce!

"Good and evil, or let's bring it down to your level of intelligence, me and not-me. It really is that simple for you, isn't it? I'll admit that keeping conscious of the multiplicities of multiverses – *ave, maria*, that's a tongue-tier – anyway, keeping conscious of all those multi's is a learned skill, hard-won, definitely. But you and your kind have sealed off so many cubits in your brain with pitch that all you've left yourselves with is a leaky boat big enough for two, and only two, of every kind. But, baby, the flood's over. You can come out of the ark now. Hell, your kind has been stumbling all over dry land for millenia."

She kept speaking out loud to herself, very out loud to herself, so Sheldon couldn't help but overhear.

"Two. Two. Rarely ever is it more than two. Existence either comes down to one, two or, on a good day, three – though it's usually just three-in-one. Father. Son. Holy Ghost. Maiden. Mother. Crone. Hecate's three crossroads. But they're all roads. Only variations on a single theme. You always have to choose. Do you see the tree or the forest? Yet a forest isn't just the same tree cloned over and over. There are conifers and deciduous.

There is grass and dirt and animals. Rocks. Streams. Mud. Shit. All this," and she winked coyly at him, "and much, much more, is a forest. And as below so above. The universe is much more than a huge black box with a gas problem. But it's always more fun to search for Euclid's point-that-has-no-part or Lucretius' unsplittable atom. Or God and Satan. Or the three little bears!

"So I'll spare you the trouble of discovering what I've learned. I'll just tell you. You probably won't grasp it. Even though, like you, it's very short and very simple. But I don't care. I'm sick of waiting for you and yours to get it. The secret is this: It's the odd that makes any of this bearable. The fourth dimension. The sixth sense. The queer. The other. But you want to pretend it away. Better yet, closet it. Best of all, kill it.

"I'll admit you're not alone. You have many friends stupider and smarter than you. Even your enemies are usually in favor of a dualistic pissing contest. Just one where they get to piss on you once in a while."

He harumpfed again. This harumpf sounded worse than the one before. He then halted his glasses' attempt to slip quietly away. He pushed them all the way back to where they'd been before he'd ever entered this madhouse.

"Please prove me right. I thought you harassed my queer children because you were willfully stupid and unaware of all the other possibilities. That you needed an easy mark to win you friends and fame. Someone to rally the wagons round now that the 'Injuns' are dead, the buffalo skinned, the forests cut down. Where to take your 'pioneers,' your 'freedom fighters' next? I know! Down the yellow brick road!

"Still won't talk? And don't give me any more of that 'I'm just a handpuppet for the lord' bullshit. Don't lie to me. You've never even had your wife's pinky, let alone anyone's hand, up your asshole."

Sheldon grimaced. He stared forward at the door. As if they were just two people – well, one person and some thing – in an elevator. He waited for the doors to open so he could get out and this creature could descend to another floor.

"Don't you ever think about what you're trying so hard to destroy – the treasures, the worlds. No, it's Ferdinand and Isabella do Spain all over again. You'd rather live without eyes than have to see anything different from yourself.

"Do you know anything about the world you're working so hard to conquer? Have you touched it, tasted it, smelled it? *¡Chinga te!* Now you've got me doing it. Shrinking all possibilities down to a lump solid enough to make a sound while it rattles around in the head. Do you know what the dirt of a fuckin' faggot forest tastes like? Before a rain? After? Do you know what a bulldyke sunset smells like? Ever listen to the music of queer sex? For a solo instrument. A duet? A full flaming orchestra!

"No. Your mouth, your mind are filled with the hates of another. No choice then. No responsibility. Just let go and let God. Or at least his legally appointed guardians on earth. What do you believe, Smalley? What do you want? If I offered you the gift of my ass, and you would be very unwise to refuse it, would you desire to bite it, lick it, fuck it, wipe it? Do you know what desire is? Have you felt it flow full on – no longer struggling to push past that rock you've rolled before it?"

He looked only at the door.

"But perhaps you do know. Perhaps I've misjugded you after all. Tell me, torturer to torturer, you *do* enjoy it. You *love* to fry up the souls of your enemy like some psychotic short order cook for Christ."

The doors flew open. The guest of honor had arrived.

Sheldon's heart fell. No men. Only more women. Even in the band. He was the only man. When would Satan arrive? He was beginning to wonder when God would. Then he stopped still and twitched. *Neither would have made Ralph Reed wait*, his inner agent whispered. Now he knew just how minor league a fallen sinner he really was.

"All these goddesses have names, many names each, none of which you'd know. Should, but you don't. So tonight we're all going by names you'd recognize. No, no. Don't get excited. There's no one here by the name of Baal or the Whore of Babylon. Inanna. I saw that. You know what I mean." Sheldon looked to where she'd turned. He saw a woman with dark skin – they all had skin darker than his – layered in gold. She was wearing the brightest, darkest blue eyeshadow he'd ever seen. She looked familiar. Maybe he'd seen her at one of his famous revival meetings.

"So I'd like you to meet Prop 67, Prop 188, Prop H, No on M, Measure 4, Amendment 2, Rider to Senate Bill..." One after the other passed by. It was worse than Halloween in the Castro. The things he'd seen those cold nights trying to save souls paled before these horrors. Maybe he'd stumbled into the lesbians' secret masquerade ball. What day was it? Was it October? Or April? Some of the women even flashed him as the old Mexican had. He grew sick.

It seemed like hours. Maybe a day or two passed. Sheldon was growing tired. He exhorted his soul to stay alert for when Satan arrives. *She's just wearing me down to tip the balance in favor of her master.*

"My, what a busy boy you've been," she said, pulling him close. The introductions were over. The band had returned, filled with a second wind. He didn't know his tito from his puente. It was all just loud horns and drums – blaring horns and pounding drums. The line of women began to circle them like a snake coiling.

Finally a man had appeared. A dignified older gentleman in a gray pinstripe suit walked towards them. Perhaps this was his bank. Perhaps it was Satan. Then Sheldon noticed he was bearing a silver tray loaded with small shot glasses. Each one burned like a fancy desert in a French restaurant. His wife would have been impressed.

"I don't think you've met the board members of the United Fruit Company." She continued to play hostess and started to introduce them. Then she changed her mind and picked up a glass. "Don't worry if the irony hurdles over your little balding head. It's a private joke between me and *centroamerica*." She tried to pat him on the head but he pulled away. "Oh, now where did the CEO go? Ah, yes, there he is. No, child," her bony brown hand was amazingly strong as it gripped his chin and tilted his head back. "He's up there."

An old man hung from the ceiling. He didn't hang heavy with death like a convict on the gallows, a human pendulum of a clock that had stopped ticking minutes before. He dangled like a gaudy plastic earring decorated with warring primary colors and bright feathers and strands of crêpe paper. Then the shock fully snuggled its way deep into the remaining marrow of Sheldon's bones. The old man had been stripped naked, hogtied with a few leather straps, painted, feathered, crêpe-papered and suspended from a mirrored ball in the ceiling like a *piñata* in the tackiest Mexican restaurant ever!

Sheldon tried not to but he kept looking. A smaller mirrored ball dangled from a shiny hook piercing the head of the old man's orange-painted penis. Sheldon winced and quickly looked elsewhere. His mouth. A red ball had been shoved in and a piece of gold shiny fabric wrapped around it and the rest of his head. Above his silenced mouth, his eyes spoke. They screamed as they bulged like the sideways eyes of red-orange-gold fish. Eyes so large and and wide and detached. As if they'd been glued on in the last few minutes rather than taking their own sweet eons of evolution to swell.

This can't be real, Sheldon told himself. *God is just testing my faith. The Lord will rescue that man just like Daniel. The Master will come skipping along the water or dance out of the conga line snaking tighter and tighter beneath the man. Just like Peter and Paul in prison, the earth will tremble, the band will stop playing, the women will stop conga-ing, and the chains will drop safely to the ground.* He'd be free. Then he, all the other old men, and Sheldon, under the command of their mighty Lord, would lay waste to Hell.

This image strengthened him. He turned to her and announced, "Whatever you threaten, witch, my final place is in heaven with my sweet lord, Jesus. Whether I go tonight or I wait until the Rapture..."

"The rapture? Oh, baby, have you got a long wait ahead of you. Girls, correct me if I'm wrong, but I heard it was scheduled to happen right after the true Messiah comes, the matriarchy is restored and Walt Disney raises himself from the dead." The music stopped suddenly for a rim shot. Then it began again. The women clucked and brayed just as he imagined the whores of Satan would.

He felt odd. He couldn't move. And he – he was looking down – down where he'd been standing before. The women were looking back. Where had all those shiny silver sticks come from?

"Sheldon, I know you have other dreams than driving the queers into the Pacific. Our little St. Patrick of Fresno, eh? And in the future, men who look and think just as you do will hold parades in your honor and drink bucket after bucket of weak beer until their faces turn the same sickly shade of green as their plastic hats. And when the party's over, all that remains is that stale smell of piss. Face it, my dear, their illegible writing's all over the wall."

The *bleat, peal, squeal* of trumpets. The *ticky, ticky, ticky, ticky, ticky* of drumsticks on metal. The *pa, pa pa da, pa pa da, pa pa dum dum dum* of hands bouncing off the taut bellies of drums. It was getting harder to hear over all the *din, da da din, da da din, da da din* of the music and the *da umpf, da umpf* of his heart. And his shoulders burned. His arms were being slowly uprooted from their sockets. He couldn't feel his legs. He was cold. He was sore and afraid.

"Your vision leads here and nowhere else. All the pain and death you will cause. For this. Choose again, *mi hija*. I can only keep my friends from spilling whatever sweet meats and other goodies that lie inside you for so long."

He tried to speak now. Anything. But he couldn't. Something was stuck in his mouth.

"Face it, Rev. You're no Ricardo Montalban and I'm no Roddy McDowell and this is no *Fantasy Island* morality play. You're in real deep shit and I'm trying to scoop you out though everyone around me keeps screaming 'Flush!' C'mon, *mi hija*. Listen to your spider grandma."

"Enough, Ereshkigal," said a shadow from the edge of the circle. "He's chosen."

"Sorry, Smalley. I tried." She shrugged her shoulders and all her leathers sighed with her. "Well, ladies, it's puritan *piñata* time!"

*

Sheldon awoke. Screaming. He'd pissed the bed.

Song of the Heretic

Jad Keres

I stroke Your soft warm skin and hear the deep hum of Your breath in my ears. I smell Your sweat and taste the salty tang of Your lips. I dream Your holy countenance and see Your immortal image in my face. You are with me always.

You call my name and beckon me to follow. I reach for Your spirit with the yearning of my flesh. You lead me to Your altar of priestly privilege and sing to me the mystery of lust and power.

I kneel before Your perfect presence and open my soul to Your carnal grace. I lay Your altar with incense and candles and burn Your glory in the wet hot night.

> *Bathe me in the juices of passion and power. Cloak me in the raiment of nobility and honor: Cradle me in*

the womb of surfeit and desire.
Teach me Your rites of passage.

I reach for Your hand of might and dominion. I fondle the grip of its hard embrace. I consecrate Your blade with a crown of fire and hail the scepter of Your earthly reign.

The dagger cuts lines across my belly. Dark drops ooze from the open wounds. I rub my hand across the red trails and soak my fingers in sacred waters.

I anoint my head with the tears of Your blood and wash my sins in the red drops of salvation. In Your name, I lick the stained fingers and drink in the nectar of holy communion.

I am the Daughter of heaven and hell. I am the Disciple of torture and joy. I am the Bitch of fear and surrender. I am the Will who comes undenied.

I stalk the shadows for the prey of seduction. I seek the night for the flesh of the beast. I slash the hide of yielding desire and I sup the meat of sweet cunt devoured.

I am the ONE.

Love and money: we strive for both, but never at the same time. Or do we?

In ancient times, the temple prostitute was beloved of the gods, the mediator between the fire of divinity and the fragile flesh of humanity. Today, she (or he) still is.

Despite the shame heaped on sex workers from all sides, the role of the prostitute remains sacred. Whores are healers of body and spirit, quick to intuit the places of greatest pain and to provide the balm. Sometimes that healing requires a touch of the divine flame, a painful cauterizing of old psychic wounds. Sometimes the prostitute becomes an exorcist, banishing the fear and humilation of her/his client's past. Today it is the dominatrix who most readily fills the role of healer. The wisest among them know their own wounds well enough to reach across the empty space from flesh to flesh and touch... themselves. The healer must also be healed.

Perhaps the time has come to re-invent the temple whore, to re-establish her honored position as priestess, mediator, and healer. These are the voices of the oracles who chart this future path.

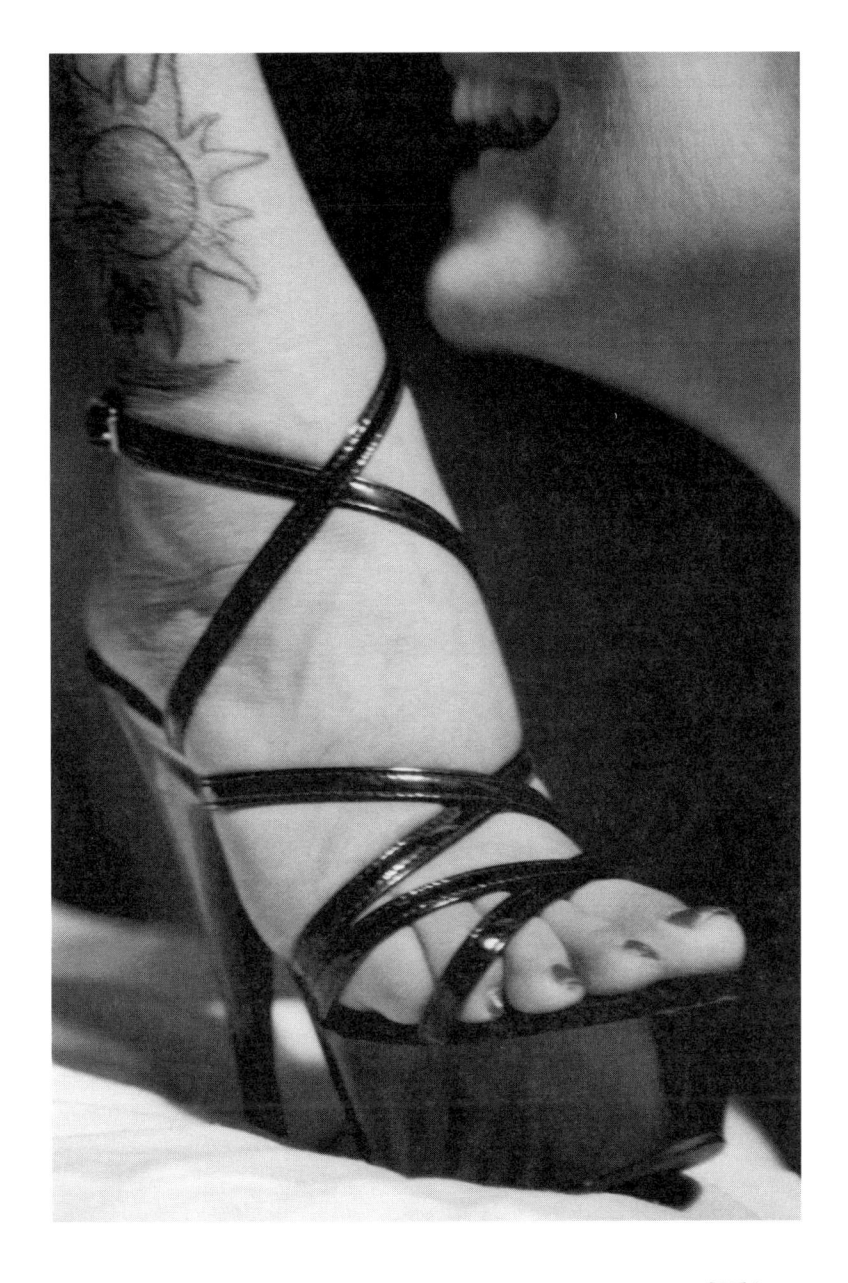

The
Sacred
Prostitute

Potato Peelings in the Shadow of Love

by Laurie LoveKraft

Gyrating to technopop they bend
Bodies shaved buttocks raised
With all the press-on features of Mrs. Potato Head
The fixed smile triggered
By eyes staring from a green paper pyramid

You are Heaven blind, stars on your eyelids
Thorns adorn your belly
But you are forest lost
Toenails lacquered red, heels stilted black

But your skin is shrunken plastic wrap
A barbed wire corset
Your body – bivouacked.
Knees bruised
Cervix tattooed
Laugh lines seared away
But I say –
I say –

Dance Girls Dance!
Arms raised bullets flying
Dance Girls Dance!

Powdered princess painted for battle
Garters of lead
Twist off nipples concealed weapons,
Your power no casualty bled

Brittle souls? They crush them
She who bends remains
Brittle souls? We crush them
She who bends remains

Asking for reparations I received
Revelations
No never ending Clinique Counter
No "Drop and fetch me a beer bitch"
But a red lit stage with parquet floor
And a pretty princess
Dancing with her life

The Dominant Woman as Priestess and Sacred Whore

Pat Califia

"One does not become enlightened by imagining figures of light, but by making darkness conscious. The latter procedure, however, is disagreeable and therefore not popular." – C. J. Jung

There are a goodly number of pagan women (and a handful of gay men and Third Gender souls) who identify themselves as Qadesh or sacred harlots, dedicated to celebrating the goddess's venereal gifts and thereby increasing her glory and power. At pagan gatherings, the line "a prostitute compassionate am I" is heard almost as frequently as the Gardnerian adage, "... all acts of love and pleasure are my rituals." In fact, these two pronouncements by female deities have pretty much achieved the status of scripture to modern pagans. While it's wonderful to see people celebrating the body and searching for a sexual ethos that is free from shame or hypocrisy, sometimes it seems to me that a woman who embraces the status of Qadesh opens herself to at least as much abuse as she does divine energy.

For example, I once had a brief and troubling conversation with a poet and dancer who does workshops on sacred harlotry. She was disturbed because male pagans (one of them her teacher) were telling her, "The goddess refuses no man." A part of her, I think, wanted to be so open and loving that she could give abundantly to anyone who asked her. But another part of her felt burned out, exploited, and disempowered by this conceptual framework. I would like to propose that this rubric be rephrased in a more feminist, gender-neutral, and Ishtar-centered form as, "No one refuses the goddess."

We live, after all, in a male dominant society where sexual pleasures are viewed askance and women are degraded, downtrodden. When a woman (priestess or no) sexually services a man, his libido and genitalia become devotional objects. There is very little hope of shifting the balance of power between the sexes or manifesting yonic divinity in that scenario. I believe the goddess would like all women to practice saying "no" to men more often. That includes saying no to one-sided "rituals" in which men are comforted, excited, and satiated without regard for the needs of the priestess who officiates on her knees, back, or stomach, focusing only on her partner's delight.

As a type of sacred prostitute, the dominant woman offers a potentially revolutionary alternative to modern Qadesh who find it difficult to escape the gestalt of dick-centered privilege in sexual ceremonies. It is a habit that is damned hard to break. I know this elucidation of bondage and discipline will offend some pagans, whom I will try hard to refrain from calling White Light Nazis, who want to worship the moon without venturing out to see what happens when she veils her face in darkness.

It will also offend some sadomasochists who have a prejudice against prostitutes and feel that any "real" or "genuine" SM encounter ought not to have a commercial basis. But it is not the exchange of money that gives many "professional" sessions an artificial quality. It is the attitude of the male client, who regards the dominatrix as nothing but a tool of his fantasies because he is afraid to experience her truth and power. This attitude is hardly unique to paid sessions. If a client is able to see the dominatrix as something other than a tabula rasa for the projection of his desires, and if she is able to operate from an authentic position of self-love and power, a commercial encounter can be as intense and transforming as any other. I know a dominatrix who tells her clients, "You do not pay me to make your fantasies come true. You pay me to receive the privilege of witnessing what some of my fantasies might be. And you pray that some of those fantasies might include a role for you." That may sound harsh to you, but I sometimes wonder if it is harsh enough to correct the great power imbalance between men and women.

At any rate, economic issues, issues of payment, reciprocity, penalties, and freedom, cannot be separated from any sexual interaction or transaction. In late 20th-century industrial Western societies, as in many other cultures, any woman who tries to control her own sexuality and enjoy it runs the risk of being called a slut and a whore. Even "the rules" girls are touched with the brush of the hustler and the hooker. They merely withhold their sexual favors for a time, until they get an offer of marriage to a high-status male. While that beats the blow-job rate demanded by most call girls, the hours are a lot longer. As long as most men make significantly more money than most women, marriage will be a brothel.

I knew I was a whore before I ever took money for sex. I knew I was a whore long before I knew I was also sacred. There's no such thing as free love, no such thing as free sex. Everything you get from somebody else comes with a price tag. Qadesh as well as their devotees need to get that straight. Trust me, it's much better to negotiate up front than it is to pretend the bill will never come due. Fortunately, the typical script for an SM scene includes a period of interviewing and negotiation that makes it easier to spell out exactly what is expected, in return for what reward.

Some pagans (and many sadomasochists) will be skeptical about the suggestion that SM can be a transcendent experience, and they will reject the suggestion that it is possible for a dominant woman to use her foresight, intelligence, empathy, and sensuality to deliberately create a scene that provides healing, transformation, and other sorts of spiritual fulfillment.

Anti-SM pagans see powerplay as thinly veiled violence or oppression; what could be sacred about that? But goddess mythology is full of examples of SM techniques being used for sacred purposes. Inanna's descent to the Underworld, where her sister Ereshkigal turned her into a corpse and hung her from a meat hook, is more severe than any consensual SM scene. When the galla, the emissaries of Ereshkigal, seize Inanna's consort Dumuzi so that he can take her place in the Underworld, it's no more or less rough than "The Surprise Party." These dramas were almost certainly reenacted annually in Sumeria. Bondage and sensory deprivation have been used crossculturally as aids to meditation, trance work, and shamanic journeying. Scourging has a long history in human religion, along with piercing rituals such as the Sun Dance and other painful ordeals. Some of the pagan prejudice against SM is nothing more than recycled Christianity, with its ban on perversion (i.e., nonreproductive sexuality). There ought to be nothing new or controversial about the idea that we can use our bodies' capacity for intense sensation to obtain consciousness of other realms.

Secular sadomasochists are often embarrassed by SM that seeks to provide anything other than orgasms and welts. I share some of this cynicism. Scoundrels often go about garbed as angels or gurus. Part of the problem, I think, is the failure of language. We are immersed in materialism. It is difficult for us to be aware of experiences or feelings that are not related to here-and-now, survival-level needs. And if we are lucky enough to experience something out of the ordinary, something magical, it often seems better to keep silent about it than allow a memory of awe to be tainted by clichés. Elsewhere, I've written about my conviction that sex (whether SM or vanilla) does not need to be justified by a supposedly "higher purpose."

Nevertheless, despite our thick tongues and jaded sneers, something ethereal and rare really is out there, really does happen, even to SM players who haven't got a clue about how to conduct a ritual and didn't particularly want to assume the mask or speak with the voice of a god/dess, or be broken down and remade into an utterly new thing. Taking spirituality away from sexuality is as impossible a chore as wholly divorcing it from romance.

First among the spiritual functions that a dominant woman can perform is the creation of sacred (i.e., safe) space. Calling the quarters, sweeping, asperging, and drawing a circle are traditionally done in Wicca to gather the ritual participants together, show them the boundaries within which the work will take place, banish mundane concerns which would interfere with concentration, push back everyday reality to make room for magic, and create a stage upon which Powers may, if they choose, reveal themselves, receive our adoration, and bless us. When a dominant woman cleans up her dungeon or bedroom, checks the batteries in her toys, sorts out and oils her whips, makes sure she has plenty of the right brand of lube and the right size gloves, she is doing the same thing.

If you cannot provide for the safety of your bottom, you ought not to collar them. This is especially important in public space, where overcrowding or rudeness may threaten to intrude upon a scene. When I top at a party or a club, I have to grow eyes in the back of my head, to guarantee that whatever mood or state of being I have created for myself and the bottom is not violated. More than one voyeur with nasty energy has gotten "accidentally" slapped with my back swing because they chose to ignore the wall I had drawn around my work. I used to invite my rowdier dyke friends to go with me to mixed parties, and we would take turns making a circle around one another while we played, mostly to protect one another from homophobic straight men who assumed any group of women ought to be paying more attention to them than we were to each other. We were functioning as a coven, even if we did not know it. We were making a safe place where women were powerful and pleasure was valued. We were doing sex magic.

A dominant woman who also sees herself as a priestess can create many different kinds of rituals. One of the most frequently performed is that of initiation – introducing someone to his or her inner erotic truth or shadow. Our culture is sadly lacking in formal instruction about sexuality. First-time experiences, if they are traumatic, can continue to cause damage long after the unwanted fear, pain, and humiliation has dissipated. Sometimes it can be healing to reenact someone's introduction to lovemaking or SM, if it was not positive, and correct the mistakes that were made or the deliberate evil that was done. Even veterans of the bedroom and dungeon can experience a need for initiation. If we are growing and learning new things about ourselves, we will constantly encounter new desires, or see familiar fantasies in a different light.

Another common SM ritual is that of the ordeal. The popularity of shoot-'em-up action movies, I believe, is due in part to a widespread desire to be a hero, to escape the grinding reality of one's job, family and "normal life" and achieve something extraordinary. There has to be something more than making ends meet and just getting by, most people secretly feel. And we all know that if you want to be a hero, you have to confront danger, take risks, and suffer pain. Even the most ordinary life contains many hidden opportunities for valor. A well-constructed ordeal nurtures the spirit of justice and chivalry. An ordeal can be a prerequisite to feeling that one is entitled to assume any new identity. For example, shamans as well as warriors need to survive their trials by fire.

Other than the ordeal, there are many other ceremonies which can mark life transitions. This may include taking a new name, donning a different sort of apparel, taking hormones, blessing new implements or equipment, or acquiring a piercing, cutting or other permanent mark to signify the change in one's status. And, of course, there is frequently a call for a formal way to celebrate new relationships or acknowledge the dissolution of an alliance.

Bondage sessions are especially suited for teaching meditation or trance work. Physical restraint and sensory deprivation can eliminate outside distractions, offer a way to make resistance palpable and yet safe, and ultimately quiet the soul. Some people are unable to learn how to develop their inner resources until they are cut off from the stimulation they routinely use to avoid looking inward. During a ritual of this type, as with all others, the power of the dominant woman and priestess to name things and give them a value comes into play. With nothing but a mummifying roll of plastic wrap and your own voice, you can take someone on a very important journey to the Otherworld, and bring them back whole, with new wisdom – if you yourself know the way there and back again.

Another important spiritual function of the dominant woman is to work with body image and gender issues. Women especially have been encouraged to feel flawed, inadequate, and unattractive. Our self-esteem is always being held hostage by a perceived need to lose weight, change our hairstyles, buy different clothes, or purchase more makeup. Even women who from the outside appear to fulfill every fashion and beauty tenet laid down by *Vogue* magazine can pick themselves apart and wind up feeling like failures. This kind of shit has got to stop! As a big girl who likes other big girls, I often find myself preaching a sermon entitled, "The Goddess Is A Fat Lady." The beauty and desirability of the Shakti exists in every woman. A priestess who can see those qualities and make another woman aware of them is doing very good work indeed.

I have mixed feelings about mass media images of the dominatrix. A part of me responds strongly to fetish apparel – shiny black latex dresses, corsets, high heels, leather skirts. Dressing up is a very important part of preparing to work as a priestess or a top. A lot of my energy comes from a narcissistic admiration of my own look, the success of visibly manifesting whatever image I have chosen for the evening. But if a dominant woman is dressing up only to please the bottom, if she finds that wardrobe limiting or uncomfortable, then it is not empowering for her to don the trademarks of female sadism. Because my fetishes include a butch aesthetic – motorcycle jackets, leather jeans, uniforms, boots, and studded belts – it is easy for me to function within a semiotic that makes me feel dominant without triggering the problematic visual vocabulary of extreme-femininity-as-cruelty. But I often have a problem analogous to that of the straight woman who gets no respect as a dominatrix if she is not wearing seven-inch thigh-high boots and a catsuit. There are lots of lesbian submissives or masochists who feel uncomfortable about femme apparel, and refuse to submit to or be aroused by anyone who wears it.

The spiritually aware dominant woman is an actor rather than an object. If I am with someone who imagines they can require me to wear femme apparel, they are going to have to deal with my police uniform; if a bottom is contemptuous of lingerie and spike heels, they are soon going to be face-down worshipping wicked pumps and black silk stockings. And I am always looking for ways to dress or appear that break up the stereotypes and clichés of pornography and pagan iconography. I will consider requests for this or that outfit, but I believe dominant women should resist any attempt by our partners to dictate this important aspect of our epiphany. Bottoms need to learn to see the divine in every aspect of the goddess and priestess.

Making gender more fluid is another potential area for the efforts of dominant women. I am especially fond of SM scenes that allow for shifts in gender identity, and in fact become more exciting every time such a change occurs. We all contain many voices, male, female, and other. In a healthy person, these are not separate personalities, but aspects of our selves. Even the most feminine woman has a strongly developed alternative reality as a man; the butchest heterosexual man can also, if he allows himself, pour his consciousness into a female vessel. There's a lot of insight and fun to be had when we become more aware of these personas. Of course, a dominant woman who wants to do this kind of work has to be in touch with her own anima and animus.

By the way, we should not assume that being a dominant woman is a femme thing. I know many butch women tops who function as priests or priestesses. Masculinity is a valid spiritual path for a man or a woman to walk. Being a man or a master also has sacred aspects. I think it is very important for the survival of the planet for somebody to create a path to male identity that is about conquering one's own shame, fear, and pain rather than inflicting these things on other people. A lot of the work I do is about validating the masculine aspects of other women's characters – their bravery, sexual prowess, physical strength, protectiveness, and initiative. I make it possible for a butch bottom to enjoy going under without being invalidated as a butch. Since I am not a heterosexual woman, I don't often do this kind of work with men, but I think manhood would be a healthier state if men could learn how to go down without being so terrified that they have to retaliate as soon as the glow of erotic gratification wears off.

As the foregoing should have made clear, dominant women frequently function as healers. We hear all kinds of excruciating secrets, and when that material is released, it becomes less toxic. Sometimes it is our job to provide a container for another person's pain. Sometimes the physical pain we inflict is enjoyed for its own sake; sometimes it triggers the release of deeper, psychic pain. Because we continue to provide loving attention during times of suffering or embarrassment, we make our partners stronger, more capable of discovery and change. The simple fact that a dominant woman accepts and shares desires that society says are sick, perverted, and unacceptable is healing.

Finally, dominant women play a spiritual role by personifying the goddess and inculcating reverence for her. Even tops who have no interest in New Agey-woowoo SM will know what I am talking about when I describe those special scenes when you seem to be possessed by something larger, wiser, and more powerful than yourself. During scenes like this, every gesture you make seems full of hidden meaning; you know things about yourself and the bottom that you have no rational means of acquiring; you are able to intuitively sense what parts of their body would benefit from what sort of stimulation; and everything you say seems like a scathing wave of poetry or an echo of deep, abiding love.

If you make the mistake of taking credit for these moments of grace, you will give yourself a bad case of hubris or top's disease. Such facility obviously does not belong to me or to you; we cannot recreate it at will. I prefer to believe that sometimes, if I am lucky, I will be visited by or channel archetypal forces that are dispensations of the goddess. I accept service as a steward or custodian for the goddess on earth. I'm a mortal woman worth no more and no less than everyone else. There is no reason why someone should wash my dishes, polish my boots, make my bed, or kneel when I enter a room. But there is every reason why all of us should serve and venerate the One who made us. A priestess represents the goddess; but we are *not* her.

This brings me neatly to the last portion of this article, a discussion about some of the problems that women face when we attempt to do ritual or magic work in an SM context. The biggest problems, for me, are related to the real-life oppression of women. It is very hard to channel loving dominant female energy in such a poisonous context. It feels to me as if the goddess is pissed off, and it is sometimes hard to know what to do with all that cosmic rage. This is where the spiritual path of the bottom comes in, perhaps. Tops don't come to the arena of SM without their own hidden agendas, traumas, and personality defects. It would be nice to encounter more bottoms who know how to function as containers for my pain; more bottoms who have been working on *their* ability to function as healers. I know this is possible because I have experienced it more than once. Bottoming well is not a simple matter of just lying there and taking it. Bottoms also need intuition. When they have good rapport with the top, they provide much more than the satisfaction to be had from flogging a bare mattress. But the education the SM community is currently providing about safe, sane, and consensual play does not usually include a discussion of these dynamics.

For the dominant Qadesh, keeping a sense of this work as important or valuable, and a sense of oneself as a dignified and serious person who has chosen a sacred path, is very difficult. How ironic it is that promiscuous women are called "easy," given the struggle that is necessary to make pleasure holy in a world that thinks it is a dirty joke. I am not complaining only of heterosexual attitudes here. Disrespect for sexually active and available women is rampant even among lesbians and feminists. When I think about how many dykes have sought my services covertly and treated me badly because I have studied bodies and ecstasy, it makes me deeply sad. A whore, sacred or sacrilegious, is not usually considered to be a fit partner for a long-term relationship between equals. I am often tempted to hang a red lantern above my door, since so many dykes behave as if one is there already. I am always trying to rebuild my self-respect in the face of constant erosion, condemnation, and criticism – much of it coming from the very same women who want me to tie them up, flog them silly, and reshuffle their psyches.

This opposition would be easier to bear with greater support. It is almost too much to do this work outside of the shelter of a temple, or at least a guild of women with a similar vocation. Unfortunately, female tops are often divided from one another by the usual lines of sexual orientation, race, and class, or we are pitted in competition against each another. It would be better for us to view one another as colleagues and sisters, shelter from the storm of disapproval and ignorance. Even if there was no stigma on being a Qadesh, I wonder if dominant women who are also functioning as priestess *can* be good candidates for long-term relationships with their devotees. It has often seemed more reasonable to me for us to form primary attachments with one another, and create our families through alliances with other dominant women.

Such connections are especially important because dominants of all genders usually need to have a place to exercise their own masochism or submission, if only occasionally. No matter how much fun it is to top, or how sexually satisfying, it is not enough to sustain us completely. We need time to let go and receive if we are going to avoid burnout. We also need to refresh our memories about how it feels to bottom so we know what we are asking other people to do for us, and how to most effectively manipulate their experience. Very few bottoms care to understand this or are able to switch with their tops without disrespecting them. A guild of dominant women committed to spiritual growth could be a safe haven for all aspects of our libidos.

There's another difficulty I hesitate to talk about, for fear of reinforcing stupid psychoanalytically based assumptions about SM being a watered-down form of murder or suicide. But the fact that Freud was wrong about a lot of things does not mean he was wrong all the time. There really is such a thing as Thanatos, an instinctual drive toward extinction and an eroticization of death. Human beings are terrified of dying, and excited by it as well. We concoct little dress rehearsals for the big moment. Some people try to control death by rushing into it; some people are in such deep denial of their own mortality that they do stupid things that facilitate their own end. One of the temptations that faces a dominant woman, especially in a world that trivializes her, is the challenge to "prove" herself by becoming progressively heavier and further out on the edge. Once you get sucked into this mode of being, it's easy to get tangled up in other people's (or your own) self-destructive dramas. Nihilistic SM is quite fashionable. I won't deny that it has its own gothic charm. But ultimately, I find this mode of topping boring. Death is, after all, the point at which everything just stops happening.

There's a valid place for work that addresses grief and mortality – our own as well as our subjects'. It's also very hard work, and many of us succumb to the numbing effects of drugs and alcohol to avoid confronting and working through these difficult facts of life. Within the SM community and within the nascent community of dominant women, we need to have more dialogue about how to separate healthy from unhealthy SM, and how to be advocates for life in a world on the brink of nuclear and ecological self-immolation. We need to do this without censoring or condemning practices or people who frighten us simply because they are doing SM in a different way. And, no matter how powerful a dominant woman might be as a healer and shaman, she needs to remember that SM is no substitute for therapy.

We also need to remember to keep a sense of humor and spontaneity about what we do. The goddess has a way of tripping up anyone who gets too pompous. And she is often pleased as much or more by the sincerity of a quick hard fuck than she is by a hollow and overdetermined rite that took months to prepare and hours to execute. The very ancient goddess Baubo can be of great help here. Her vulgar dance, rude remarks, and exposure of her own genitals made Demeter, who was mourning the loss of Persephone, laugh and take pity on the world she had sentenced to death by drought and famine. Baubo is as holy as the more formal, well-known, and grand great goddesses.

A woman who accepts a vocation as a dominant is in direct opposition to feminine conditioning. Women have been taught to have a horror of taking sexual responsibility. We are supposed to wait passively for others to court us, endure whatever sort of physical attention they give us, resent their clumsiness without correcting it, and demand economic rewards in exchange for this benighted existence. This system is obviously unsatisfactory, but it is impossible for one individual to change it completely. A woman who wants to control her own sexuality and have pleasure in her life is in a dilemma similar to that of a working wife and mother. As women, we don't want to give up our hard-won right to an education and a paycheck. But without a more radical social transformation, these "rights" can easily become variations on female oppression, entitling us to nothing more than a dual shift as homemakers, childrearers, and wage slaves. For many women, a partner's suggestion that they start topping during sex just feels like just one more selfish and unreasonable demand on their time and energy.

Even the dominatrix is always in danger of being turned into a servant. It often feels easier to follow the path of least resistance and focus on other people's needs than it is to discover our own. The SM community could address this problem somewhat by emphasizing that any negotiation for a scene should have as its goal the satisfaction of both partners' requirements, and acknowledging that bottoms as well as tops can be unsafe, unskilled, or dishonest players.

When we are high on the admiration of others, it is easy to feel as if SM is all we need to make ourselves feel good and make our lives run smoothly. But the exercise of sexual dominance in an SM context is not enough to make women free. An infusion of feminism completely changes the nature and character of practicing SM – as does an infusion of spirituality.

I do not always approach my scenes as a Qadesh. But I want the values which inform my spiritual practice to regulate how and when I play. The possibility of using SM techniques for ritual purposes has opened up many new experiences for me and made it possible for me to make connections with people I otherwise would have missed. It's still fun to simply trounce a good, heavy masochist just for the hell of it. But a bottom who comes to me to work on a spiritual issue as well has added another level of trust to the game, and a whole other dimension of intimacy and insight to our play. There isn't a lot of written information about how to safely and effectively perform on that level, and it's my hope that this article and the book it appears in will spur a discussion that will create such a body of knowledge. If we build the temple, She will come.

Cleo Dubois

Interviewed by Carol Queen

I was born and raised in Paris, France, in a very fanatical right-wing family, and went to a Catholic girls' school, run by nuns, until I was 15 years old. I had a very strict and twisted French Catholic upbringing. My family was severely dysfunctional. My father suffered from alcoholism and my mother's entire life's work is ultra-right political beliefs. I did a performance piece a couple of years ago about what it was like to be raised (or rather, suffocated) in a French pro-Nazi environment. There was a part of the French population, a small part, that collaborated with the Germans during the war. My mother and her family totally bought into that. She married my father because he was also a follower of this ultra-Christian Right, racist belief system. My family imprinted me with military images, guilt and secrets. My mother still writes part-time for a French fascist newspaper. My father died; I made peace with him in the last months of his life.

I was also a survivor of rape. When I was a virgin, almost 18, I got gang-raped. I had been trained to "keep myself for the right man," and to repress any sexuality. I got no support from my mother when I eventually told her of the rape. She simply said it was my fault for acting sexy. I lived in fear, denial, and violence in those days because of my father's alcoholism and my mother's political tyranny, which was really taking over her life.

In 1969 there was a general strike in France. That strike gave me a sense that everything I had been taught was lies, and that I could reject it all and have hope for a different life. So I went into the street and fought with the students, and threw rocks at the cops, and read Sartre, Foucault, Genet, and Proust. I became a monster by my parents' standards. Shortly after the whole "Student Revolution" failed and everybody went back to work – it was early '69, and the hippie movement was still happening in San Francisco – I just said, "This is it, I'm leaving."

My escape was very romantic and naive. I flew "to San Francisco," and made "sure to wear some flowers in my hair." I had no marketable skills, spoke almost no English, but was determined to make a new life for myself. I tutored French "au pair" to kids of upper middle class families in Marin County and did a little sex work, very innocently – I worked in a massage parlor. And men asked if I did French, and me believing they were asking me if I was French and saying yes! But I kept on rubbing their backs.

In 1975 I went back to France and travelled to Egypt, where I fell in love with belly dancing. When I returned to the States I supported myself performing in Arabic clubs on Broadway. It was sensual work, and that was powerful for me. I looked at belly dancing as an art form. I maintained my body for myself, nobody touched it, and I was an unattainable object of desire – or so it seemed to me! But in my private life, there was something missing. It was 1976, a time of many affairs, a time of sexual permissiveness. I enjoyed going to sex parties, orgies we would call them at that time, and it was fun, but there was something at the core that was not working for me. I felt unfulfilled.

One evening several years later I got invited by a lover, a Renaissance man who was into explorations of all kinds, to a salon that took place in The Gorilla Grotto bookstore. There, Kat Sunlove did a presentation on SM. She was one of the first in the Bay Area to teach classes about it. All of a sudden I got it that this was something for me. It was instant light, lit up in my heart and my cunt and my head. She mainly talked about the difference between nonconsensual violence and consensual erotic play, and gave a whipping demonstration with her submissive partner. My own exploration in SM started immediately. Things that flashed in my head were the power of those images that I had been raised with, military, fascistic images, power images, dominance. I saw that there was a path that was really different but used some of the same elements – control, fear, intensity, but in the opposite way, with "turn-on" and consent. And it was like an instant revelation: Yes, that's what I have been missing!

And then I remembered instances when I had a very sweet lover and I used to figure out ways to piss him off and have these screaming fights, so that he would lose it, and he would actually hit me or slap my face, and he'd be on his knees apologizing, and I'd get all excited to see him like that and then we'd have great sex. I got it: No, that was really not the way to play with this energy! Yes, this was very hot, powerful, and very sexy but carried on all this guilt about violence and abuse. And there was no clear agreement, no negotiation, just manipulation.

I joined the Society of Janus, an SM education group that Cynthia Slater founded in 1974. I was going to Janus programs and demonstrations and really getting involved in the discovery of consensual sadomasochism and bondage. Fakir Musafar was an early Janus member and was giving all these strange programs, about body play, piercing, and so forth. I attended all of these, so the concept of body ritual came in immediately to my awareness of SM and felt right to me.

My personal affinity with men was with gay men. Gay men liked me because of my "Frenchness" – and that I found them so sexy! My lover Mark was bisexual, and both of us were coming out into SM – I met him at Janus. I got welcomed into some inner circles of SM gay life, where I got a priceless education and healing, in clubs that no longer exist, like the Catacombs, the temple of fist-fucking and SM, where the feeling of family and wild abandonment filled the room. The first time that I entered the Catacombs I was very scared – I was the only woman there. The space had been opened to women by Cynthia and Pat Califia, but neither of them were there that evening. But after a couple hours I was home. I recall being fisted to a big orgasm where I was crying, laughing, coming, and screaming "I'm home," all at once.

There were a lot of ecstatic experiences in my life. And then AIDS was amongst us. It felt like all of a sudden my friends were getting sick and dying – the carpet got pulled out from under me. I got scared, broke off with Mark, and the Catacombs closed, all the clubs closed, the Folsom district changed over to art and straight clubs and entertainment, and I went into a very intense depression, though I didn't know it at the time.

What kept me going through that time was professional dominance. I knew that Cynthia did professional SM, and I asked her for advice. In 1982 I quit working at the Sutter Theatre, which was the last burlesque theatre in San Francisco, and had started doing part-time dominant work at a studio. But the woman who owned it had no respect for her clients. She saw them as foolish tricks. She was not really in "the scene."

I really believed in SM as a valid psychosexual exploration. I loved it! So I put all the money I made into equipment and within a year my friend Sybil Holiday, aka Mistress Cybelle, and I opened up an SM dungeon. From the start I was self-taught, bottoming or submitting to gay men in sadomasochistic play, and immediately turning that experience over and becoming the dominant, topping straight men at night. That felt natural to me. I was proud of my work. I got repeat clients, men I could look at straight in the eye, intelligent, middle-class men who kept coming back for my services. And that kept me going, that I had a talent and a gift. It gave me courage.

I did not compromise myself in professional dominance, which is one of the reasons why I have not burned out, but to the contrary, am enthusiastic about teaching others to actualize their "kinky fantasies." I knew that for me, with my background, I had very clear boundaries around men touching me. So I asserted myself as a sensual, sadistic dominant, with a heart and feelings, but did not do body worship scenes, where I would be touched or kissed. That would have a tinge of prostitution for me – oh! and that was not okay for me. It's taken me a long time to come to the understanding that I need to be supportive of the work of prostitutes. I used to not accept or understand the concept of the Sacred Prostitute. And I regret in the past I've been judgmental. It's not wrong, just because it is not for me. I still can't really say that I do sex work, 'cause I still don't think I do it. I call what I do psychoerotic work.

For me, an SM scene, whether it's a private scene with a loved one or a professional scene, is still a special, intimate, ritualized experience. I look at SM and bondage as vehicles for transformation – a place where surrender, intimacy and big pleasures can happen, where I can really give, take, or receive – and that is all sacred! The roles I like to play involve control games, turn-on, and intense sensations.

When I do a good scene I feel good and connected with my bottoms. Now I'm teaching more couples, and my focus is expanding. In the past it has been mainly men – who desperately seek a place of surrender, of not being in charge. I understand the need for that place, so I can take them on those journeys where time stands still. The erotic energy is like the gas in the car, it makes the engine run, so my work is really erotic but it also has a real overtone of exchange of power. I know I'm in charge and I am aware of the responsibilities I take. To have this private situation where a total stranger can trust me is wonderful.

I do a lot of bondage. When I'm tying people up or doing sensory deprivation – blindfolds, hoods, gags, mummification, in suspension – and intense sensation, they can resist for a while, but when they surrender, they can fly. It can be set into little scenarios, like helpless captive or Mistress/slave, but what makes it work is that trust and communication be there between the top and the bottom: one who's willing to take charge and be really present and the other one who's willing to say, "All right, I wish to surrender, to give you what you want or receive what you will give me."

I really value bottoming and switching in my private life. It's an integral part of what I need. I learn a lot every time I "go under"; it's an inner journey. I also cherish the bonds I have with people I bottom to –

it's a whole sense of sacred trust. I mean, we're looked at as perverse people, and I look at us as people who are able to honor various aspects of each other's sexuality in sacred space. So my sense of being a "pervert" is really opposite from the judgments of the uneducated.

There are archetypes that sometimes come through when I'm playing, and it can be with friends, with lovers, with clients – the Woman Warrior or the Woman Healer come through me, the Great Mother or Kali – and I'm not just Cleo Dubois being a sadist, I'm a channel for this larger energy that gets me out of my head and guides me to be like a craftperson, taking people on journeys, like a pilot on a wild aircraft. That's the magic of the work. It empowers me and turns me on, and it also empowers the "bottom."

Some people can really fly with beautiful, really intense whipping. I remember those instances where I'd be holding the whip, a special single tail whip I have, whose handle is made of a cobra, and all of a sudden my energy space changes and I feel I'm going to cry; I have tears in my eyes and I know I'm going to strike like a total goddess. This archetypal mother or warrior is going to strike that person and it's really going to hurt and it's so beautiful. Those who seek that experience sense it at the same time as I, and we don't need to talk about it – it's like I'm bottoming and topping at the same time, energy moves through me and guides me. I'm really empathic with the submissive and then I strike and it's like fire. And there is a beauty and a magic there – this ritualized violence has a peaceful, loving intent.

We can welcome big archetypes that are divine energies, but we can also play with those human models of control and oppression that are part of our society. In "play realities" we can cleanse these roles of their offensive qualities. Compassion, turn-on, and dominant sadism are words that fit together in my world!

I get remarkable feedback from people who don't necessarily know that's what we're playing with. They say, "I've never felt that way, this was incredible, I was high and everything fell into place and my heart opened!" I've done work with many Vietnam vets where they get in a real quiet place, and it's scary for them. I remind them that they can trust, and that big boys can cry here. You know, this is the most intense work that I do. I don't want to sound too scary, I do fun work, too, but if I stumble onto those shadow places there is no avoiding them. I just become really compassionate and human and keep being there, whether I stop the scene and hold the person or push them through it gently – or not so gently.

SM for me is about sexuality, growth, healing, and intimacy, about spirituality, but I realized that it wasn't enough in itself. Going into psychotherapy and searching for who I am helped me integrate those images and the healing that SM experiences gave me, let me take them out of their separate boxes. I'm sad that SM work is not really understood. If I could work with therapists, if we could consult back and forth, I think it could be good work. The way it is, the healing is there for the client, but if they don't have a therapist who's SM-positive, or they don't tell anybody about it, the tendency is to keep what they're getting from the SM in one place and the shame about their "perversity" in another. I do encourage people to gently come out to their mates if possible.

I value very much the counseling I received around my abusive background, from two different professionals who both understood that SM is a path for me. My therapy, my queer community, and my partner helped me with my own integration. It's mainly about going inwards, facing my fears, my shadows. So my work as a sadistic dominant is now more solid and nurturing. That comes with getting older, too.

I have to accept that so far I have lived my life "on the edge," and I acknowledge that the fear is there, but I do not let it take over. Many here have done work to make our lives as "perverts" more understood. As humans we need to trust and feel universal love, to accept one another's sexuality, and we need big pleasure that connects us to the Divine. Which is what a spiritual experience is to me, that you experience the stuff yourself, with your body, like some other cultures do in their body rites.

Specifically I am talking of Malaysia where I went last year to this big festival where people have all these piercings, with objects like bells sewed to their skin, dancing themselves into a trance to their gods and goddesses. I have done this sort of ritual many times. Fakir and I were in the same community for a number of years, and eventually we connected and became partners and mates, and I experienced with his help a lot of body rituals, which in the cultures they came from do not have the stigma of sexual perversity.

We as SM people can see how these rituals and SM play connect. You may not be bottoming to a single person, but you're bottoming to this universal love which is also very present in your own body, and Bliss is then tangible. These are ancient shamanic practices that are archetypal adventures – that take your body and your spirit to the same place. They don't separate your body and call it sinful and bad, from your spirit and call it honorable, like we do in this culture. It's like going into the darkness to see the light. Actually in the Tamil Hindu religion of the Thaipusam Festival – the one we went to Malaysia for – there is a belief that there cannot be light without darkness, so this path is a path of darkness to the light.

I just returned from a wonderful trip to London, where I spoke to art audiences about body ritual, SM, and dominance and submission – focusing on trust, intimacy, intense sensation, bondage, and ritualized play between people as the vehicle to healing, reclaiming, and inner exploration. I received an enormous welcome from English women, who felt validated in pursuing their own "kinky" body explorations.

Now I want to guide people who are getting titillated by the visual aspect of fetishism which is everywhere. They buy SM equipment and fetish clothes and feel that there is something more to it, but they don't know how to get to it. If I can help empower women, I think I am doing a good job. I know a lot of men who'd like to come out to their partners about their need to bottom. I'm sure a lot of women fantasize about either being dominant or being dominated but keep it strictly in their private fantasies.

Now that all these visuals are out in the culture, I feel there is a real need to share knowledge about what's underneath them. Around safety, of course, and skill level, but also around the increase of intimacy that one can gain by revealing one's sexual fantasies – of power, the forbidden, helplessness, sluttiness, being taken to the limit – all that stuff that makes us really hot. Safe play that may look unsafe from the outside, because this stuff always looks different than it feels; fantasies that include non-monogamy, playing with people of different genders and sexual orientations, voyeurism and exhibitionism.

I wish to encourage women to take control erotically. It does not come easily for women to allow themselves to receive or request pleasure. I also want to honor our vulnerability and the beauty of surrender. It sounds scary, but pushing limits can be done very gently, just asking for a little bit, and topping can be very fun and joyous and seductive. Not just strict and stern.

The roles we choose to play in SM and D/S can bring out hidden parts of ourselves, like our inner child, inner free slut, queen of our private world, or inner girl if we're a man, and in that playing there can be healing, self-discovery, and great pleasures.

Working with couples, the male partner is often the one to initiate, because of the way this society is. The woman might come a little bit reluctantly and be more afraid. If I can help her look at her fear and talk about it, that's good. Her partner usually wants to be dominated, and he's trying to push her to get dominant. I show her that there might be something in there for her, help her center and feel her power so she can stop thinking that it's going to be a lot of work to please him, and rather get in a place where dominance is an adventure of empowerment and erotic exploration for her. It's about letting herself feel strong and in charge. It's not about acting out stereotypes of the professional dominant, like in Hollywood movies and SM porn.

In a safe situation, the woman can start feeling strength and turn-on by taking control. I have noticed that a lot of women can be sadistic, but they don't feel safe in that space because they do not know how to craft that energy. Doing SM is not the same as lashing out at somebody. I have given women a soft whip and the first time they flog their partner they go full force. If I'd given them a hard whip, the guys would be screaming. So it's not that the energy is not in us as women, but we have to learn to build it up, to seduce with it, and then to let it out and savor it.

I have spoken to a lot of males who have tried to share their desire with their partner but instead of approaching it in a loving, subtle fashion, like "I'm having the fantasy that it would be wonderful if you'd tie me up a little bit and..." they might say something like, "I have this intense captive fantasy and I want to go to this SM store and buy all that equipment. I want you to tie me up, put a hood on me and use all that equipment I've seen in the SM catalogs!" They do not put themselves in the place of someone who is new to those games, reveal their secret gently, and help their partner feel comfortable with it. They want the whole thing – totally overwhelming their partner. Especially if they have seen professional dominants on the side for years. They think that coming out to their wife is doing the same negotiation they do with a professional, and that just doesn't work.

Also, showing up with $2,000 in bondage equipment on a first play date might be a bit much! A more successful approach might be to share the desire to let go of control, rather than the explicit description of the kink. Sharing the desire to be taken and the wish to honor and adore the woman they want to bottom to is a far more important message to communicate.

Often two partners want to switch. And I certainly understand that. Men who want to learn to be dominant erotically are also seeking help – it has been my delight to see that they have some of the same concerns as women. They don't want to hurt their partner: "How do I know she's going for it?" Simple things like just asking if she is okay might not come to their minds, or noticing how she breathes, looking into her eyes, or what her body language is. They want to tie her up and bring her ecstasy or give her a chance to be the bad slutty girl she always wanted to be. But they don't know how to do it.

It takes being centered, wanting to make it work and being willing to work at it with your partner. That's what I've learned in my own relationships as well. Going too fast and too far can take years of slowing down to get back to where you wanted to be in the first place.

These adult games can be very powerful. And we must be safe and responsible when we explore intense realities. We're talking about taking emotional risks with each other, as well as creating this huge, wonderful intimacy. Stop if it's not working, not hot, or if it feels too scary for the top or the bottom. Re-establish "straight time" – it's not time to get angry or blame yourselves, but just be present for the other. Roman Polanski's "Bitter Moon" is a good study in not knowing when to stop.

I look at an adult letting his/her vulnerability shine as a gift. I handle it gently. I do not humiliate a submissive about showing themselves that naked – I tell them how beautiful they are in that space with words or touch.

Having come so far, and having learned so much through my explorations of SM both personally and professionally, I have begun to teach on a more formal basis by opening the Cleo Dubois Academy of SM Arts. My vision for the academy is to have workshops that are a couple of days long, and have several couples attend who have similar interests. There is a lot of empowerment in being seen playing in a safe environment, and people could share information. So far it's been mostly one couple at a time doing private, guided play in my dungeon. I offer an introduction to SM and bondage, with negotiation and demonstration, guided play for partners, tailored to their specific needs and skills, guided play for unpartnered dominants with my female and male submissives, and I am giving more public classes in leather stores and for adult organizations.

You know, I feel privileged. I'm in a very good, interactive queer community with much diversity, where we are freer with each other than most people know is possible, with respect and understanding, and I love to see these options open up for more and more people.

Calibration

Maude Wolff

Preface

She was a vestal virgin at that time. Indeed, at that time she was chaste, though not by plan or desire. She had served well the friends who came to her hearth. For them, there was always food and wine and laughter. And when they left, sated, loneliness for her. Some had touched her body, fondled it. Occasionally, pleasured it, but they always stopped short of true consummation.

She walked up the stairs slowly. It was the traditional day of atonement; the day the god of Abraham and Isaac decides who will be written in the book of life for the year. Although she no longer subscribed to that religion, she felt that she had atoned her entire life. But for what it was unclear. Each stair brought her closer to her desire. It sounds so trite, of course, but it was true. At a deliberate pace, she climbed to the new life that she knew was hers.

The woman at the top of the stairs was attractive in a quiet way. Both women were of a similar build. She felt a soothing sense of familiarity: I have touched a body such as hers and pleasured it deeply, so like my own it is. That body won't lie. That body can be trusted.

She walked down the long hall with the woman of the house. They engaged in comfortable small talk. Her new friend opened the door to a room and bade her enter.

She entered the dungeon slowly. Not like dungeons of folktales, this room was immaculate and beautifully outfitted with rope sculpture and solid wood restraining structures. Her new friend brought her a cup of tea and left her alone with her thoughts.

Although the day was fiercely hot, the dungeon was cool. The air was clear, like the air in the high mountains. The room was calm. After looking around, she sat down and folded her hands. Peace engulfed her.

Many years before that, she had meditated in a thousand-year-old monastery. Though exhausted from the journey, when she entered the ancient meditation hall and prostrated herself where countless others had, she felt a sense of total calm and renewal. Now, for the first time since she left the land of snows, she felt that same peace again.

The journey home had begun.

Reconciliation

The journey home had begun. A different kind of journey. The currency of the realm is desire. Its value increases as its name is spoken, its intricacies explored. A treasure chest awaits not the one who conquers, but the one who surrenders.

To walk through the jungle of the senses. Not trooping or despoiling, but walking deliberately, slowly. Walking with beginner's mind: noticing colors, textures, vitality, and fecundity. Everything is alive and resonating. Even the quiet has voice. Like walking meditation – in breath, out breath, in breath, out breath. Regular at first, yet quickening. Quickening almost imperceivable. Quickening with desire.

She had wanted this journey since she was a child. She had tried many times to begin. Each time, when her senses were exposed in full daylight, she panicked and ran when she saw her shadow. Each time she ran away, she died a little inside.

Now she walked in the full force of the sun to embrace her shadow. She was not without fear. But something inside her had gnawed the restraints of fear until there was no other path to follow. She began the journey to reconcile the warring forces that tore at her core and sabotaged her every small victory. After so many false starts, she had begun her journey to reconcile spirit and desire.

Beginnings

She said to her teacher, "How will I know my limits?" The teacher told her, "Like calibrating a fine instrument, we are looking for the pivotal point where pleasure and pain intertwine, transcending ordinary experience. As your cravings give rise to experience, your limits and desires will expand. Activities that you think you cannot tolerate today will soon become your comfort zone. Each time we are together, we shall spend a few minutes re-establishing our calibration.

"Now to begin. You will not be in physical bondage just yet. However, you are in bondage as you stand here before me. The restraints that hold you are infinitely stronger that any rope, leather cuff, or chain in my collection. It is the force of your desire, your need to experience and understand. Is this correct?"

"Yes," the student replied. "I am here because I want to be here. Here because I want to feel alive inside in a way I've never known, only imagined. My intuition tells me this is the way, but my conscious day-to-day awareness is afraid."

The teacher continued, "As I was saying, I have omitted restraints because I want to see your unrestrained reactions. You may ask questions. You may use your safeword to stop the proceedings if it becomes more than you can bear physically or psychologically. You may ask for more. I may or may not fulfill that request. Remember, you are here to explore, to work with your fears. Only you know the difference between your true limits from those barriers you wish to overcome.

"Remove your clothes."

The student removed each article of clothing, folding it neatly and placing it on a chair. The room was silent, except for the rustling of fabric.

With the removal of each article of clothing came the lessening of her outer-world persona. Her "blending-in" defense was rendered impotent as her tailored suit, silk blouse, and undergarments were laid to rest on the carved oak chair. To her surprise, she felt less embarrassed naked than she had imagined. Her overwhelming desire to be explored left her spirit as naked as her body. She faced her teacher, head bowed in respect.

"Walk to the center of the room." She did. "Spread your feet apart shoulder's width. Leave your arms at your side and hold that position." The student complied.

Lesson 1

The teacher circled her student. At first she touched the student lightly, as if measuring her for a gown. Then she stood behind her and cupped the student's head in her hands. With strong fingers she explored the student's skull beneath the thick black and silver hair. She moved her hands down the cranium to the neck. She held her hands securely encircling her student's throat. Sensing panic in her student, she said, "Your first lesson is trust. Just as I want the inside of your throat for my pleasure, so I want the outside for my control. You can still breathe. I won't take your breath. Put your left hand on your diaphragm and your right hand beneath it. Concentrate on your breathing. You will learn to trust me and yourself."

The student moved her hands in compliance. She began to breathe in a slow way, as she had learned many years before. She was aware of the pressure on her neck, which seemed to pulse with her breath. She realized that the panic rising in her chest caused a much deeper constriction than her teacher's hands. She knew that her self-imposed bondage was greater than any her teacher could ever construct. This internal bondage was the bondage from which she wanted to escape.

The teacher understood the exchange of power. On a rudimentary level, so did the student. It was the foundation on which they were building. Over the course of lessons the student would exchange her self-imposed bondage for that which her teacher created; exchange self-imposed pain for the exquisite pain of the dungeon. Over this sacred period of time, she would learn the lesson of simple surrender, the joy and wisdom it can bring.

The first assignment was encircling her neck: trust. Trust herself. Trust her teacher. Breathe in and feel the power of her teacher's hands pressing on her neck. Breathe out and feel those same hands supporting her against her vulnerability. She felt the panic in her chest, then named it energy without the label of panic. Felt the transition from the edge of panic to the edge of acceptance. A small journey, whose progression she didn't fully understand: edge of panic to edge of acceptance. This was her introduction to the pathway and the process she would follow countless times to come. She relaxed and accepted her teacher's hands as a necessary part of her musculature.

The teacher removed her hands. She stepped to the cabinet and removed a leather collar. "You will wear this today. It will remind you of my hands on your throat, remind you of your desire for surrender, remind you of my control." So saying, she tightened the collar and fastened it snugly.

Lesson 2

The teacher asked her student to clasp her hands behind her head. The action lifted the student's head, raised and lifted her breasts. The teacher watched. Then she walked behind her student and studied the lines of her back. It was a strong, well-muscled back with broad shoulders. The teacher caressed it with her fingernails in long, vertical pathways, admiring how easily her student marked. The marks lingered, exciting the teacher. It would be a pleasure to dance a flogger across her student's shoulders. But that would be later.

The student arched her back ever so slightly as the teacher explored her ass. Watching her response, aware of a quickening of breath, the teacher knew that the key to her student's surrender would be here. She studied her student's ass. It was a sensual ass: enough muscle to know the difference between tension and relaxation, enough padding to take a thorough beating and beg for more. As she ran her fingers slowly down her student's crack, the student began to move slightly, trying to draw the teacher's hand in deeper. The teacher was delighted to discover such a hunger. How exquisitely exciting to demand and receive surrender from so deep within.

The teacher moved to the front of her student. She lifted the student's head in her hands and looked in her eyes. The student demurred and looked away. The teacher slapped her lightly on the cheek. "Look at me," she demanded and slapped her again. "If you are to be my student, I must look into your eyes. If you are afraid to meet my eyes, then this work that you crave is too dangerous. Look me in the eyes or leave. I do not work with cowards."

The student met her gaze. While their eyes were locked, the teacher began caressing her student's breasts. First the right, then the left breast, the teacher pinched a spiral pattern into each one. Again, the student squirmed and received another light slap. "You do not have my permission to move, stand still. If you stand very still while I finish, I shall let you change positions."

The teacher took a breast in each hand and began kneading as if there were two mounds of dough to be shaped into round loaves. She moved to the nipples, pinching them, pulling them, and twisting them, testing her student's perseverance. To her student's credit, she endured admirably. She was visibly aroused: her breathing and the beads of sweat in her cleavage gave her away. But she remained steadfast. The teacher was impressed and aroused.

"You have earned a rest. You may sit on the floor in the corner by the cabinet. You will please crawl there." The student dropped to all fours and began to crawl away from the teacher. "Stop," the teacher said. "I want to see more of you. Put your forearms on the floor and spread your legs, so I can see you better. The hallmark of a good student is one who makes a gift of her vulnerability. Not only must you open yourself to me, but for our work to be truly successful, you must rejoice in doing so. Soon, it will become second nature."

The student crawled into the corner taking care to move slowly, deliberately exposing her private parts. After so many years of trying to be invisible, this deliberate exposure was at the same time demeaning and deeply exciting. While building her career, she struggled to be rewarded for her brains, not her body. She divorced her body and its pleasures, a corporate eunuch. Now she was reclaiming her desire. She felt herself blushing all over – ashamed and proud of her arousal. She felt her cunt getting wet. She hoped that her teacher would notice. Her spirit soared at the thought. When she reached the corner, she positioned herself into half-lotus, sorry to be once again self-contained.

Memories

She watched her teacher move about a low table. The table was padded in black leather. The teacher placed a small pillow in the middle of the table. Then she covered the table with a quilt. The quilt was of rich autumn colors, deep greens, maroons, sienna, ivory and rust with an aubergine border that was almost black. The teacher fastened the quilt to the table. She noticed a puzzled look on her student's face.

"Yes, black leather is the stuff of fantasy and I am covering it. I am covering it for many reasons. You and I are dealing with fantasy, certainly. But on the deeper level, what we are doing is as real as everyday life, as real as this quilt. Other people use this table, the quilt isolates each person's experience. Your journey is an inward one, like the retreat of the forest in autumn. What appears to the world as the leaves fall is bareness. What the trees experience is quiet renewal, a preparation for the next period of fertility. The leaves that fall nourish the earth and the tree digs deeply for that nourishment. Think about the metaphor. You may draw strength from it during our time together.

"There is one other reason for the quilt. Just as I must care for the ropes and whips and all the things in this room, you must care for the quilt while you are my student. If it is dirty, you must wash it. If it is torn or fraying, you must mend it. Quilts have a life of their own. Like a lover, they require care. If this task is too traditional for your liking, dress and leave."

The student didn't move a muscle.

"Good. I think you will find that caring for something that is outside of yourself yet intimately connected with you will enhance your commitment. The name of the pattern is Memory."

Lesson 3

The teacher moved nearer the student. She took an implement from a hook on the wall. It had a leather handle and a doubled-over strap of black leather about three inches in width. The teacher held it in her hand. She said, "I want you to crawl around the perimeter of the room to the table I've prepared. Crawl slowly as before. Keep your head down. Begin."

The teacher took a step backward as the student took one forward. She studied the view, noticing the wetness around her student's cunt. She felt her own excitement mounting. She tapped the student on the ass with the strap. "Stop, you are going too fast." The student obeyed. "Rest your forehead on the floor. Rather than be in such a hurry, I think you should savor what I have for you. Keep your legs spread and your ass in the air for me and don't move."

So saying, the teacher dragged the leather strap slowly from the top of her student's crack to her wet cunt. Down then up. She slapped the strap lightly on the student's asshole. The student arched her back. "Such a hot ass. I think I must cool it down a little." To a rhythm only she heard, she began to beat her student like a lovely drum. She began slowly, stroke to the right cheek, stroke to the left, each pair of strokes gaining a degree of intensity across the virgin skin. "Are you cooling a little, my hot one?"

"I don't know how to reply," the student said. "I am frightened. I am excited. I am terribly embarrassed about being excited and that makes me more excited. It hurts and I want it to stop. And when you stop, I want it to start again so badly that I feel I'll burst if it doesn't. I don't understand all these conflicting desires and sensations dancing in my mind and on my skin. I don't know exactly what will please you, but I want to please you. And, I want to feel alive."

"Very well, bottoms get wishes granted, too, sometimes. It will be my pleasure to continue spanking you as you crawl. Be a good little girl and crawl slowly. Remember to keep your legs apart so I can watch your charming cunt and asshole. They are so inviting. Tell me about the last time they were visited. Was the guest a tongue, a finger, a cock, a toy... perhaps multiple guests entered? How about a little drumming to accompany the story, like raconteurs of old. I shall keep time on your ass. That should keep you in the spirit of the story. Amuse me and I shall reward you."

Memories

The student thought about the last time. "I suspect it will be a disappointment to you. It was to me. I had met a very effeminate man. Because the best sex I've ever had in my life was with gay men when I was much younger, I thought this man would be similar. This man flirted with me. I decided to call his bluff. It had been five years since my last lover, a woman.

"After several aborted tries we managed to get together at my house. Involved with someone else, he was hesitant about being unfaithful. I told him that if it would be traumatic we could stop. He laid there with his eyes closed for a minute or two and then began to touch me very tentatively. I touched his ass and he jumped. He then asked me if I liked to be touched there. I said yes. He said that perhaps some day we could try having sex there, if I didn't mind. I suggested this was as good a time as any. He rather half-heartedly agreed. I rolled onto my stomach. He got on top of me and smeared cunt juice for lube. Then he entered me. It hurt a little, mostly because I wasn't ready. As soon as I adjusted to his being inside me, he lost his erection. End of story. No, not end of story. I then spent the next half hour convincing him he was really okay. After he left I was in a state of total frustration, so I went to a store and bought several toys. I also began the investigation that led me to you. End of story. But at least, I got an idea what I am looking for."

They had reached the table. The student was stationed at the foot of the table awaiting further instructions. The teacher was lashing a series of light-to-moderate figure eights across the student's ass and upper thighs. It was one of those magical moments when the balance of openness and sensation was just right. The student felt she could stay there forever. The teacher was intrigued with the student's honesty and with her intense level of frustration. It would be a challenge to unlock it.

Lesson 4

"Climb onto the table and lie on your belly." The teacher positioned a pillow under the student's pelvis. "This will keep you properly presented to me. Again, I am not going to bind you yet. I want to see your unbound reactions. Now after your story, I suppose we should start where your unfortunate friend failed. I must dress for the occasion. While I am doing that, I want you to think about what it will feel like to be full. You have told me this is what you want and I want you to anticipate it. I want you to tell me that you want me in your ass." The teacher reached for gloves and donned a double pair.

The student hesitated.

"What, you don't want it any more?" the teacher asked. "What do you want, a game of Gin Rummy? Are you wasting my time? Tell me what you want."

Quietly, the student said, "I want to spread my legs as far apart as I can and I want you to look at my cunt and my asshole. I want you to..." The words stuck in her throat.

"Yes, you want what? Do you want me to look and not touch? Do you want more impotence in your life? How about an enema of political correctness, about three quarts? Maybe a thorough caning. We aren't playing a thousand questions. You must take the risk to name your desire, otherwise you may never claim it." As she was speaking, the teacher took her cat-of-nine-tails from its place on the wall and began lightly whisking it across her student's tender ass.

"Does this ass of yours want me inside it?" the teacher said, striking it a little harder than she intended.

"Yes," came the quiet response. "My ass is yours, do with it as you will."

"You should be a little more careful of your request, it may be my will to cane you to a bloody pulp, to penetrate you beyond your liking, or to sit with my knitting and ignore you. Be specific. What do you want?"

"I want your hand in my ass and I am very afraid. Please don't tear me. You can hurt me, but please don't tear me."

The teacher stopped whipping her student. She laid a gloved hand on the welted ass and gently rubbed the welts. She bent down and kissed the small dimple at the top of her student's crack. "The top and the bottom serve each other. I take you where you want to go, but you have to have the strength to tell me where it is. I'll be your tether on your journey, but you have to hold on with some part of your will. I watch your responses, subtle ones of which you are not aware, to gauge my next action. It is true, I love hurting you. I love pushing you. But I do not want to damage you and I damn sure don't want you to damage yourself. You must tell me if it starts to be too much. You cannot abnegate your responsibilities as a human just because you are a bottom. Terrible form. Be advised, banishment is the punishment for neglecting your responsibilities! I'll send you away." And with that, the teacher slapped her student on the ass and walked to the side of the table. She knelt down and looked her student in the eyes. "OK, look me in the eye and tell me what you want."

"Please, will you put your hand in my ass and if I can't take it, will you stop? And if you have to stop, will you still let me come here? I've fantasized about this for so many years and never found anyone I would trust enough to even say the word. I'm afraid of failing, so afraid."

"Kiss the whip, I think it pounded some sense into you. I would be delighted to explore your ass. Let's see how far we can go. I want to feel my hand in there. If not today on the table, perhaps some other day in a sling. I trust you followed my preparatory instructions and cleaned yourself well inside?"

"Yes," the student replied, blushing deeply.

"Did you continue until the water ran clean? Did you enjoy it?" asked her teacher.

"Yes and yes," her student whispered. "I thought of you while I did it."

"Good," replied the teacher. "Next time, I'll control the flow."

"As far as failure," the teacher continued, "the only failure that I recognize is a failure to speak openly and negotiate bravely. If you are willing to be honest and to claim your desires and to enjoy them fully, then I shall be pleased. Trust is a two-way street. If I can't trust you to tell me what you want and describe your journey, how can you trust me to take you there? Sensation is a tool to surrender; it is not surrender itself. It is perhaps a more exciting road than the one followed by yoginis in frozen caves. But it is still a road to a very similar place. Remember that.

"Now I have a small request." She put a condom on the whip handle. "While I begin to explore, I'd like to watch you suck the handle of the whip. As with all we do, start slowly and work thoroughly. And I shall do the same."

She walked around the table, looking first at the sweet face licking the end of her whip and then at the very red, elevated ass, awaiting her fingertips. She reached for her most viscous lubricant. She poured a large amount of it onto the student's ass and began applying it to her asshole. She massaged slowly around the outside of the hole, rimming the anus with her gloved index finger. She then rolled her finger in the creamy lube and began to apply pressure against the anus.

Her student groaned, then apologized for making noise. The teacher responded, "No, it is important to make noise. I want to see and hear and feel you respond. Let the sensation evoke movement and noises. Don't force them, don't fake them, don't try to figure out what you think will please me. Just ride the sensation and respond, and don't forget to suck the whip handle. I do enjoy watching you get fucked in the mouth." Her finger rested in the band of the first sphincter. Her student groaned with delight and raised her ass, greedily taking the finger into the second sphincter. The teacher rotated her index finger and slowly began to insert her middle finger. It went in immediately, swallowed by gently rotating thighs. With her left hand, the teacher poured more lube. She moved her ring and little fingers into position under her middle finger and inserted them. Though her intention was to go slow, she found that they, too, were welcomed immediately. She fell into the age-old fucking rhythm, fucking with her right hand; teasing with her left, and watching her student come alive with movement, with sound, and with passion.

Physics

Timing is such an odd phenomenon. Specifically, I am thinking about the intersection of a raw desire and the desire fulfilled. Like an atomic model with desire at the core and attempts at fulfillment circling; whizzing past, but not colliding.

And then, one day it happens. Desire and fulfillment collide, obliterating one another in the process. Energy, in the form of intense heat, is released.

Odd, that once my mind began to function again, this was the image. Probably it was poetic justice for all those times I sat in physics classes with a vague desire I could not name. Now I know how to describe it. Your hand in my ass was the collision of desire and fulfillment.

The Sacred Prostitute and the Three Kings: A Most Radical Faery Tale

MATAKLAR

Once upon a time, in a far away land, there lived a prostitute. But She was not your typical prostitute; She was very special, for She had dedicated Her life to goddess worship and in doing so became a sacred prostitute. Her brothel was the Temple of Desire. Her altar radiated divine female sexuality. But She was not your typical sacred prostitute. As high priestess, She had a particular vision and a mission to seek out balanced energies to taste, test and take unto the Goddess for Her divine enjoyment and pleasure. She received visitors for this sole purpose.

One day, three visitors approached Her temple professing to be kings from the East. In their lust they travelled quickly and argued who would be first to experience Her pleasures. The "biggest" king intimidated the others with bullness and physical strength – so they agreed to go in order of diminishing "bigness." When they arrived at the temple gate, the prostitute confronted them disguised as a fearless guardian.

"Who comes to the temple?" She demanded, "and what do you want?"

The biggest king stepped forward and delivered the introductions, announcing that they came to see the sacred prostitute and had brought gifts of great value.

"Be seated in the courtyard," the guardian instructed, "and wait until you are summoned."

After a while, a drum sounded and a voice rang out like a cymbal calling the third king to enter the temple. The visitors looked at each other in confusion, for this defied their agreed-upon protocol. The third king shrugged, then humbly walked through the doors, recognizing great honor in being chosen first. Upon seeing the radiance shining forth from the altar, the king immediately fell to the floor in adoration. The prostitute gazed down upon the king, body and soul, and saw a true balance of female and male energies. She also looked upon the gift, saw that it was given freely, and determined that it was precious indeed. Then She welcomed the king and the gift into the temple sacrum and judged that they would serve the Goddess well together.

Later that day, a drum sounded and a voice called the second "bigger" king to enter the temple. The visitor entered the doors and hesitantly announced the gift. Searching through the brilliant light for the prostitute, the visitor continued to move forward... when a voice commanded, "Kneel, you fool! Where are your manners?" The visitor fell to the floor and apologized profusely, not quite understanding what was happening. The prostitute gazed down upon the visitor and the gift and found an inkling of what She was searching for. She reached deep inside the king and tested the presence of female energy, then spoke unto that part of being that She had touched.

"This will require much effort on your part. The Goddess will demand sacrifices and offerings. You will have to stretch to please Her. It will not be an easy task. But the rewards will be great. Do you understand and consent to this?" Afraid to look up at the prostitute, the visitor nodded and promised to make the required effort. The prostitute looked upon the king and the gift, and judged that they would *potentially* serve the Goddess well.

Much later, a drum sounded and a voice finally called the "biggest" visitor to enter the temple. Angry and insulted at being summoned last, the visitor strode through the doors with head held high, and loudly proclaimed the preciousness of the gift. Seeing the light of the altar but not the prostitute, the visitor strode confidently forward...then suddenly fell to the floor, stunned by a tremendous blast of energy that first brought stars to the eyes, then total darkness.

"Where are you?" the visitor screamed. "I want to present my gift, but I can't see you."

The prostitute gazed down upon the visitor and the gift and determined that both were worthless. "Poor little 'big' king," She laughed, "you have not brought me anything of true value. Your 'bigness' is simply a mask to hide your insecurity and lack. You came seeking to capture and possess the Goddess to make up for your own lack of female energy. How dare you pride yourself as superior to the others when your energy is entirely unbalanced?" She continued, "Your salvation would require a difficult rite of passage involving the sacrifice of your puffed-up hollow ego and the acceptance of female energy into your being."

Still blinded, the visitor protested, "But why should I have to make such a sacrifice?"

"You do not *have* to do anything. The Goddess only accepts gifts that are freely given. Go now."

"But I have travelled far to partake of your beauty," persisted the visitor.

"Then you shall continue travelling in your lopsided vanity." And with those words, the prostitute sent the visitor off to wander blindly around the world, deluded by the myth of "bigness" – like Diogenes, but without a guiding light or a supreme purpose in life.

After the temple gates closed, the prostitute priestess cleansed the space of "bigness" and looked kindly upon the two kings who had chosen to remain in the service of the Goddess, one still trembling awaiting trials and tests to come, and the other purring contentedly at Her feet.

The moral of this story is threefold: 1) Beware visitors who bear false gifts, 2) Energy balance is essential for well-being, and 3) *Never* underestimate the power of the Goddess!

The most ancient faiths acknowledge the wisdom of the gendered body. To this day, traditional Jews pray that their virtuous acts on earth will be mirrored in heaven, so that God and His Presence, the Divine Feminine or Shekhinah, can be reunited. As humans make love on the Sabbath, so is the Divine brought into unity with itself. The pre-Hebraic goddesses of the Near East, Ishtar and Isis, harrowed hell to preserve the bodies of their consorts, because only in union with them could the earth flourish. The disembodied, invisible god is a recent – and impoverished – invention.

The body does not lie, but the truths it tells us may seem strange indeed. Sometimes the union of masculine and feminine that we project onto the gods, we neglect in ourselves. Entering into the service of the goddess, we find ourselves transformed... into ourselves. Inner realities – phallus, womb – do not always manifest in flesh and blood, and so we create them in ritual and carry our metamorphosed selves into the light of day.

Some women look into the goddess's mirror and see the face of the consort, both strong and vulnerable. Men, too, can see this image, or the shimmering face of the goddess herself. What we see is what we know to be true: our bodies become the site of our worship, our own temples and groves. We create them from our native soil, and sometimes with rock hewn from a distant quarry. The result is a space where we come face to face with our own truth.

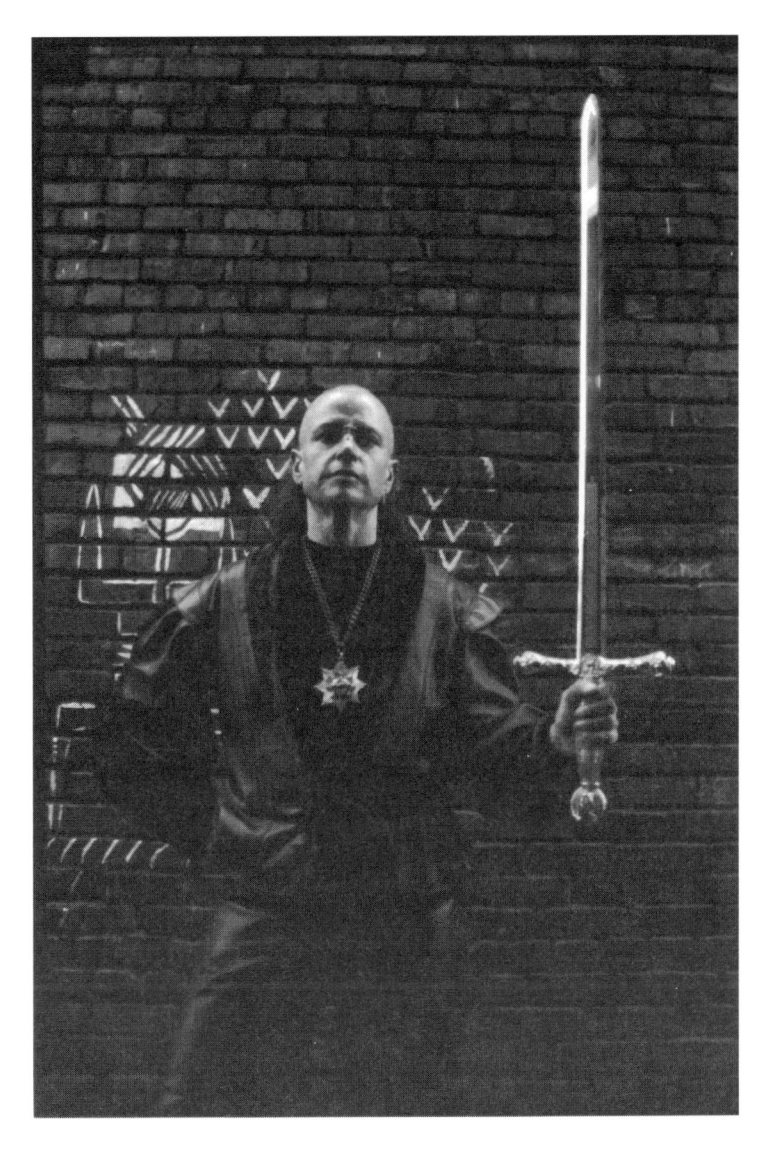

God/dess:
Engendering
the Divine

Tellers of Fortune, Dealers of Fate: Dark Goddesses and Unmanly Men in Northern European Traditions

Bill Karpen

> 'I don't mind mocking the gods,
> For I think that Freyja's a bitch;
> It must be one or the other—
> Odin's a dog or else Freyja.'
> — *Njal's Saga*

For many centuries, unmanly men in the northern lands of Europe have made sacrifice to, muttered prayers to, incanted spells beseeching, danced in ecstasy for, seen visions from, and adorned themselves as the goddesses of that region. These are the goddesses who make the snow fly in the heart of winter, who gather the souls of the dead and lead the spirits of the unborn on their midnight sojourns, who teach the arts of seeing to humankind, who weave the grisly sinews of fate.

Somewhere the unmanly men got lost in the stories that have come down to us, the fairy stories of how things used to be. The storytellers no longer understood the tales of the men in skirts who seek visions or work strange forms of magic or speak with animals and the spirits of the woods or the dead. They did not fathom the role these men had in the tales, and so they changed the stories to make sense once again, only without those men. And then again many stories must surely have been forgotten because they no longer made sense without such men in them.

Sometimes one sees glimmers, such as the boy who cooks and tends house while his brothers go out to hunt in the forest. He it is who coaxes secrets from his mother and befriends the sister they have sworn to slay. He is the one whose arm remains in the shape of a swan's wing, harking back to a time when such transformations were the mark of such men as he. And then there are the tales of masked boys dressed as beautiful and ugly Perchtas and other masked figures wearing cowbells who beat each other with sticks at Carnaval in order to bring abundance. Or even the tale of the little one who finds himself in a family of ducks until he discovers those graceful and powerful beings called swans, finding as well that he is one of them.

She it is who scatters gold or else pitch. She is the beautiful or else the ugly Perchta. Each one chooses which face She will show. One daughter chooses gracious Hulda, the kindly grandmother; another daughter chooses maleficent Hulda, the harsh mistress.

Once she rode the earth astride a horse of three legs. Half black half white she was, above beautiful and fair, below dark and rotting. It is said that she would appear outside the dwellings of the gravely ill to ease their pain, one way or the other. They say that for those between life and death, Hel would ease the way.

The man in the moon looks down from his perch. Some say he carries a bundle of sticks. Some say he kidnapped a boy and a girl carrying a pail of water. Some say that he comes down to the earth on nights when the sky is dark, that he wears a skirt. The man in the moon watches, watches everything: the fish as they swim through the sea, the people in their beds or their various nocturnal perambulations, the wolves as they wander, the owls as they hunt. He sees all. He watches over the people of the night who see what others do not. He sees the other side of the dream.

In that space between the old year and the new, Hulda or else Perchta or Holle or Hildeberta or perhaps simply Berta rides with her wild host collecting the souls of the dead. In that gateway between one year and the next opens another gate between the lands of the living and the lands of the dead. Furious is her company, witches and man-wolves, night hags and enchantresses, spirits of the living and spirits of the dead. Through forest, field and fen, over hills and down into valleys they roam, shrieking and keening the long night.

It is said that bands of these creatures wander from place to place, peddling their trinkets and their art, which is the telling of fortunes. Swathed in scarves and skirts and jangling with strings of tiny bells, these men, such as they are, ride into town singing and shouting and banging on pots and pans. They sing loud and bawdy, tempting the boys and taunting the girls.

But when the cloak of darkness covers the landscape, people make their way to the strangers' camp a little way outside town to hear them tell the fates' decree for their newborns or what the harvest will bring. A roast of mutton or a loaf of rye in the crook of their arms, they arrive at the camp and set the food on the table for the seers. After a while, the wandering visitors once again begin to sing, but the songs are different now, eerie and mysterious, calling to the spirits of other realms. And they begin to speak, sometimes only one at a time and at others several of them, forming a graceful cacophony of visions, twining together and slipping apart.

She sits, legs dangling over the stones at the edge of the well. From one hand dangles a spindle as the other hand twirls it, spinning the flax into thread. She does nothing but spin, and she has done nothing but spin for some time now. The fibers of pale flax twist together into a fine strand. Raw are her fingers as now they begin to bleed. Seeing the first trace of blood on the flax, a gasp escapes her lips and the spindle escapes her grasp. She climbs stumbling down the walls of the well until her head knocks against stone.

She wakes to find she is by a roadside. She starts to walk and soon comes to an apple tree laden with fruit. Its branches droop with their burden, and she hears the tree ask if she would shake the apples from its limbs so they will not break. She approaches the tree, taking its trunk between her hands, and begins to pull. The branches start to swing up and down and the apples one by one begin to drop, bouncing this way and that, to the earth. After a time and many apples have fallen, the tree gratefully thanks her. She walks onward down the road, and after a bit by one side she finds an oven full of baking bread. The bread cries to her to take it out for it will burn otherwise. And so she does, laying it by the side of the oven to cool, and continues once again on her way.

But now the sky begins to darken as the sun sinks behind the hills. The wind picks up and chills the girl, for she has no cloak. Still she walks on. Just as night sets in and the calls of night birds begin to resound from the echoing hills, she sees a light through the trees and at last she comes to a cottage. Much relieved, and yet fearful of who may dwell within, she climbs the steps and knocks on the oaken door. An old woman appears, long of tooth and long of nose. She invites the girl in and tells her she may stay with her if she will but clean the house, being careful to shake the featherbed until the feathers fly like snowflakes. So the girl does as Mother Holle bids, making sure to clean the house till all is shining and clean and shaking the featherbed till the feathers fly like snowflakes. Mother Holle in turn treats her kindly, never speaking a harsh word to her and keeping her well-fed. The girl is quite content for a time to live with Mother Holle, and yet there comes a time when she begins to feel homesick. Soon it becomes unbearable, and she asks Mother Holle if she may return home. Mother Holle graciously assents, thanking her for her labors, and tells her that she will show her the way. She leads the girl to a door, hands her the spindle that had fallen into the well, and bids her farewell. As the girl passes through the doorway, she finds herself covered in gold and only a little way from her house.

Her petty sister is not so lucky.

With misshapen lip, monstrous thumb, and fearsome toe, these three old women spin. One lip, one thumb, one toe in the world of human beings, the other in the realm of the freakish, the grotesque. They spin flax, yes, and other less mundane threads. Unsightly and even ghastly they may seem, though for one lazy girl, their magic with flax was a godsend. Your wedding, they told her, you must have us to your wedding. What they did not say was that this gift would save her fingers evermore from touching thread.

Once one would say that one was growing swan's feathers when a strange foreboding came over one. Many stories are told of women who would don a swan-shift or else a swan-ring or swan-chain so as to take the shape of a bird. In some tales these women would tell the future, and they would always bring good fortune to their loved ones. Most often they would travel in threes, and sometimes one of them would be obliged to remain in human shape by him who stole her shift or ring or else her golden chain.

The sound of rain falling on the canvas overhead. The voice asking what the goddess would say. The intake of breath as the spirit of the seer leaves the body and another takes its place. Pleasantries first, but then something else. Do you know how much trouble you are to cause? She is the stirrer of strife saying this. Strife was stirred when the women took back their power, she says. And so must you. For complacency is the closest thing we have to sin. Eye to eye she stares at the one who posed the question: Complacency is the closest thing we have to sin. Complacency – the fear of stepping to the edge of that which is known, of striding out into the darkness beyond the pale of the comfortable and safe. The fear of obliging others to do the same. The fear of moving stagnant waters to flow, for flow necessitates penetration as the waters stream through one's being. Unknown powers entering, potent and uncontrolled, coming through the channel opened to them and coursing throughout. Desire becomes manifest in the directing of the current. Staunching the flow leads only to rot, the body dead before the heart stops beating. Complacency is the closest thing we have to sin.

It is said that among a certain tribe, the Naharvali by name, there existed in times of old a temple that was dedicated to twin gods called the Alcis. At times these gods took the shape of snow white swans or else of strong-necked stallions. Deep, deep in the woods was this temple, more sacred still because of the men who served as priests there. These men were decked out like women, they say, but the stories do not say what they mean by this. Perhaps they dressed entirely as women, with gold and silver brooches pinning together long robes of linen carefully dyed with madder or else with walnut husks or wode. Maybe they wore bracelets and rings and wore their long hair braided and pinned up in the manner of noble women. It may also be that they wore skirts but underneath them the breeches of men, that they wore tinkling bells after the fashion of the unmanly priests of Freyr. Other stories, if we are to believe them, say that such men were especially skilled in the arts of seeing visions, of casting curses as well as blessings, of foretelling the future, arts that were otherwise scorned as mere women's magic.

They wandered the roads, these women, travelling from farm to farm, village to village. Mostly there were but three of them, although at times either seven or else thirteen. Some folk called them the fates, others seeresses or fairies and at times the wyrd sisters. One story tells of them spinning through the night the threads of a newborn child's fate. Another tells how they came to the house of a newborn boy, how many came to witness the blessing, how the fates were offered food and drink and gifts. The first two sisters bestowed great happiness upon the babe. The third, however, pushed off her seat in the crowd, rose up in anger and cursed the child to live only so long as the candle beside him should not burn out. The first sister quickly pinched out the candle and instructed the mother only to light it on the last day of the boy's life.

There are many other stories as well of these women who wander from place to place telling fortunes. There is of course the tale of Briar Rose who by the curse of the thirteenth fairy pricked her finger on a spinning wheel. And it is always a curse that flows from the lips of the last fairy or fate or wisewoman, though the reason for her malice is always different.

In the stories of the first of these unmanly men, men called them cowcunts of sorcery, bitches of prophecy. Not always well loved were they, for some deemed them less than men and therefore contemptible. Among some peoples, they were drowned in swamps, and there was one, Eyvindr by name, who was tied to a sea rock and overcome by the tide. There was Ragnvald Rettlebone, who was burnt or else drowned along with eighty more. Unloved they were, feared because of their unmanly skirts, their uncanny powers, their unfettered lust. They straddled the abyss between man and woman, animal and human, society and wilderness, life and death, safety and danger, spirit and flesh, blessing and curse. Murder was the only means of controlling these creatures, of fixing their ebbs and their flows, of making them safe.

She roams the outskirts of civilized places, for those who have created these places do not know her, do not understand her, and there is no place for her within walls of the known world. The walls bar one from being whole. Women are like such and such; men like so and so. But she is not one of their women, and the men who follow her are not their men. Even after all this time, these fey men remember that she is the mistress of some other realm, a realm where they have a place.

Even from across the hills one can hear the raucous cries of battle – the clash of sword on sword, the thud of axe on shield, the death songs of the wounded and dying as metal cleaves flesh, the wyrd chantings of fey women weaving the fates of warriors. Grim is the sight of the battle; grimmer still is the sight of these thirteen women with their broad loom of slaughter. Bloody entrails form the warp and the weft, severed skulls serve for weights while swords, spears, and arrows make up the frame of the loom. These strange creatures chant over this canvas the names of the slayers and the slain as bloods flows from every thread.

She who goes between the warring tribes, who thrice withstands the spear's blade, who thrice withstands the flame's tongue, she who desires penetration. Freyja, at the stillness of that maelstrom, guides its flow. She, sowing the seeds of discontent, of yearning, starts the waters to motion. She rides the tide of lust, the clash of life force with life force, the spray of brine, the spark of iron on iron, the dizzying flow of blood.

Eager they are, and eager is she. Eager to absorb the essence, the juices, the power of those who come into them, just as she. Eager for pleasure, eager for the touch of unseen flesh. Unseen knowledge flows through these unmanly men, these cowardly men, these skirt-wearing, bell-jingling, shrill-throated men. She, as they, open to the streams of wisdom coursing through the cosmos, is penetrated by visions, drawing them through her form, and spinning from them her web of power.

There is a whole troupe of them just emerging over the top of the next hill. One never knows for certain if one will see them – you must happen upon them or else they upon you. They could be heard even before their heads rose over the crest, though, their jingle bells jingling in the crisp midwinter air. In some parts of England, they are called mummers, and in others guizers or plough boys or whatever else. No one seems to know when or how they started making their annual pilgrimages, although they have been doing so for centuries.

All of them are dressed in odd costumes, white with ribbons tied about their shirt sleeves. Either they wear masks or tall tall hats covered with beads and looking glass or maybe plumes and strips of old clothing hanging down; perhaps their faces are painted black. One or maybe two together are disguised as a horse. Perhaps there is one dressed all in tatters, shreds of cloth hanging down looking like some scraggly beast. There is surely one of the men dressed up as an old woman with a long nose and carrying a broom. Sometimes they call her Besom Betty or perhaps Mother Molly or Dame Jane. Maybe too there is Old Hind-before and Jack Finney, or Beelzebub with his dripping pan and club in hand. There are certainly two men and maybe more with swords by their sides. One may be St.

George and the other either the Turkish Knight or Turkey Snipe or Swish Swash and Swagger. And of course there is the Doctor.

At any rate, as they get to the house, a knock is heard at the door and they boldly tumble in. One begins with a few rhymes, and then one of the fighting men and then the other. They challenge each other and come to blows, one by and by striking the other down. One of the players will call for a Doctor, and in he marches, lately come from Italy, Spittaly, France, and Spain. He can cure the itch, the stitch, the palsy, and the gout, and by some trick or another manages to cure the fallen man. Then come the rest of them: perhaps it's Beelzebub dressed in a frock, or Big Head with his little wit, or Little Jack with his wife and children. Each makes a few rhymes, at times about houses thatched with pancakes or straight crooked lanes, at others about magpies walking about in pattens and drowned in dry ditches, or leather bells a-going without their clappers. Then the players start to go around asking each person in their small audience to put money in their hats or pans or baskets in return for luck in the coming year. And off they go, the whole lot of them, off to another house or farm or village, jingling their bells as they go.

Hers is the heart of winter, when all things slumber. Hers is that which is out of season – the souls not yet born and the souls whose time has passed, green herbs when all about lies snow. In the stillness of this darkest season, she clears away the dead branches to make way for the green shoots of spring.

The call went out in the morning, and one by one, or by twos and fives, the faeries, as they are called, began to create things for the procession. Painting lipstick, rouge, and sequins on faces, and hanging gowns, skirts, and cocktail dresses from bodies and poles to be held high in the air, they invited the spirits from realms far from this one to join them. They rubbed charred sticks on limbs to make them appear as bones and made masks of coarse paper to resemble skulls. Tambourines, bells, pots, rattles, drums they gathered to announce their intent. With paint or markers on broad sheets of cloth, they remembered the names of their dead. Some laid flowers and dried leaves, garlands and strings of stones, images of goddesses and gods on the altar to the dark goddess to be carried on their shoulders. As the sun dropped behind the high ridge of the hill, they began to coalesce in the clearing beside the barn, drumming and chanting and making last-minute preparations. And then they began to form a long column by the beginning of the road, the drums and chants becoming louder and stronger, the altar rose and drifted first this way and then another until it found itself in the midst of the procession. And then the whole dancing, rhythmically pulsating mass, tall poles draped with dresses, faces painted or else eyes gleaming from behind masks, banners billowing in the evening wind, began to flood onto the road.

Bibliography

Andersen, Hans Christian. *Eighty Fairy Tales*. Trans. R. P. Keigwin. New York: Pantheon Books, 1976.

Brody, Alan. *The Mummers and Their Plays: Traces of Ancient Mystery*. Philadelphia: University of Pennsylvania, 1969.

Carnavals et Fêtes d'Hiver (Carnavals and Festivals of Winter). Paris: Centre Georges Pompidou, 1984.

Chambers, E. K. *The English Folk-Play*. Oxford: The Clarendon Press, 1933.

Davidson, H. R. Ellis. *Gods and Myth of Northern Europe*. New York: Penguin Books, 1990 (original publication by Pelican Books, 1964).

de Vries, Jan. *Altgermanische Religionsgeschichte (Old Germanic Religious History)*. Berlin: Walter de Gruyter & Cie., 1970.

Ginzburg, Carlo. *Ecstasies: Deciphering the Witches' Sabbath*. Trans. Raymond Rosenthal. New York: Penguin Books, 1992.

My Life as a Consort

Robin Sweeney

The Indian import store where my household buys supplies for rituals is run by a very nice woman named Mira. She recognizes me, and shows me some of the statues of Hindu deities she has for purchase. Her store is stocked with incense, beads, jewelry, fabric, and clothing from India. She also has one of the best selections of Hindu devotional statuary in the area. I am looking for a statue of Hanuman.

I am attracted to Hanuman, the Protector and Servant of Ram. I love the idea of a monkey deity, and the stories I read about Hanuman delight me. He moved mountains, literally, for his Lord, Ram. Ram recognized the godhood of his monkey general, and made him a god in his own right. Hanuman is typically depicted in his helmet, carrying his mace. Mira has an affordable statue of Hanuman, his palms together in a prayerful position, which will fit nicely on the hodge-podge altar I keep at home. I have a Hindu corner of my altar, next to my drum and in front of the space I put my car keys and pocket watch. I want Hanuman to be there.

I take him to the counter, and prepare to pay. She looks at me, and then at the small image of Hanuman.

"Very odd, you know. Hanuman is not usually a symbol for women. Very odd. Women like Lakshmi, or Sita. Not Hanuman. He is a warrior, you know, and very masculine. It's odd for a woman."

I smile, pay, and agree. Yes, very masculine. Uh-huh. Very odd, that's right. I'm an odd duck, and an even odder dyke. And I am one weirdo spiritual being, too.

Too butch, too weird, too difficult to categorize.

I was too butch for the semi-permeable membrane of the lesbian community at the college I attended. I was too weird for the gay politicos I knew. Even when I found San Francisco and the leather community there, I was still a little strange. There was more room for my oddness, certainly. There were people who liked me both despite and because of my butch identity and my intensity, but I am still odd.

When I started searching for a spiritual home and community, I discovered I was just as odd there as I was in the queer and kinky worlds.

Buddhism was too somber for me, when I first found it as a teenager. Everything is too somber for a fifteen year old, and sitting zazen was no different. However, the ability to sit still and attempt to keep my mind clear was a valuable skill, as I rocketed my way through my teens, drinking and drugging and hating myself. (I giggled through my first mummification scene, years later. I had found that place of stillness and calm and imminence before, through sitting meditation. I knew how to count breaths and wait for the magical pictures in my head to happen. Sensory deprivation just made it easier.)

Later, I began a sort of half-assed attempt at some sort of magical practice, to give some of the parts of myself I had buried under alcoholism a chance to breathe. My limited psychic abilities – to ward, to do some hands-on healing, and to make people answer questions that I hadn't asked out loud – began to wear on me as I stopped drinking. (I wonder now, if there had been anyone in my life to point out that this was a real, and understandable, phenomenon, if I might not have spent as much time drinking as I did? Would I have believed someone explaining that I wasn't crazy when I was an adolescent?) The limited resources that I found to answer some of those questions helped some, and if a magical path or tradition had been available to me, I might have followed it.

Instead, I got pretty good at divination, bought some fascinating books and a pile of semi-precious stones, and still had no focus for my spiritual search.

Then, I found a niche in the Episcopal Church. That was extremely confusing for me. I was raised with no religious tradition, and came of age as a queer who was always – and often rightly – suspicious of organized Christianity. Finding myself belonging in a place that I never imagined myself to belong, in a religion I never thought I would be comfortable in, was downright weird for me. It was an incredibly safe place to experience unconditional love within the structure of faith. For a while, it was a home.

I love the Church, with its sense of tradition and ritual, the structure and community I can sometimes find there. But I eventually found myself uncomfortable with the single-minded approach to faith that Christianity offers, and it was painful for me to be as non-traditional as I am in a very traditional religion. Even though the church I attended was gay supportive, the clergy candidates they sponsored were all mainstream gays – not kinky, not weird, not gender oddities, and all coupled off with life partners. I'm queer, I'm a pervert, and I'm non-monogamous. I didn't fit the parameters.

There is no place for my magic in the Episcopal Church.

And what is that magic?

I am a woman who does men's magic. I am a female-bodied person who assumes typically masculine roles in magical rituals. I guard the perimeter, I drum the rhythms of the circle, and I am the Consort to whatever Goddess I am with. I balance the polarities of the people I make magic with. All the dark magical creatures I have in my life, who are women or female or queens or goddesses, I answer as clearly as the sun breaking on the horizon of Solstice morning.

I don't walk the path of the twisted trickster of gender, I more stumble along. While I like to cross-dress as a man, and have enjoyed the times I have passed as a man, it is more about being able to conjure up what is the essence of masculinity for me. This hardly feels like a path at all, but if I keep walking, I guess it will be. The best hiking paths are built that way, with stumbles and mistakes and veering around prickly bushes.

My magic is a Daddy thing. I nurture and care and fuck and tease and provide a masculine balance to my partners. It's a Daddy path, it's boy magic. It's the creation of the sacred wet spot. I have a dick, here, somewhere in my psyche, and it's much more powerful than any other part of my body, or any other magical tool I have.

My magic wand, you ask? Right here in my pants.

I had no idea that there was a Goddess there for me to find and serve and care for, until I looked around and realized that all the women I knew and loved were avatars of some sort of Goddess. The time I spent thinking there was some force out there that would come to me through the correct prayers, rituals or spells was, in reality, around me all the while.

I've fucked Bridgid and heard her rip me open, from deep inside her body, as she came on my arm – in a language I can only guess at as Irish and old and known in my bones. Poetry as clear as any I am compelled to write echoes in my head from her, and all I can do is fuck her in gratitude.

I've had a woman, who is a little boy, beg me as her father for forgiveness. "Please, Daddy! I'll be good!" as I beat her. I've granted her absolution, and showed her that faith in a forgiving father is possible, and close. Seated on the right hand of the father, indeed. Be Daddy and pass on the ways that I have found to be masculine and powerful and not an asshole, this is part of my magical job.

I turn over my power, my strength and my place in the universe, and let my lover – who is a follower of Kali and sometimes becomes very much like her deity of choice – take over. She takes over my breathing, my body, and my blood. She rides me, and fills me, and scares the hell out of me. Sometimes the best I can do is lie still, and let her have her way. Her way involves me walking through all that terrifies me, and embracing it, and thanking her, as Mother, for letting me have this connection with her. I know why Shiva smiles in all those pictures of Kali dancing on his chest.

I work the runes. They first came to me in my dreams when I was very small. They have been the way I have left my mark, when I needed to leave my name in a special way since I learned to write. The marks that I started using to leave my name appeared in my hands from the first commercial set a lover gave me, and I knew I had found part of my answer. I hear the whispers of the Elder Gods, and know that there is another man gaining knowledge for me from hanging himself in a ritual. It only got weird when I started reading more about the runes, and ran into a whole bunch of stuff about how women weren't ever really supposed to work the runes. More stupid, sexist garbage that made me feel like the magic ways I worked couldn't be real.

I long thought there was no place for me in a goddess-based tradition. It's one of the problems with the way that paganism is presented – a goddess is always a woman, and a god is always a man. It's heterosexist, and confused the hell out of me, when I started searching for a pagan direction to walk in. I'm female, yes. I've wrestled with my demons to get and stay with that definition, thanks. I finally had to decide that I wanted to be a different kind of woman, more masculine than not. I didn't want to be a different kind of man, which I feel like I would have been if I had decided to take testosterone and transition. And I'm not a different kind of man, today. My strength comes from being raised to be one thing, and making magic as another.

I'm staying in the body for this length of time, complete with all the parts that are jarring and sometimes alien feeling for me. But when someone blesses me as an aspect of the Goddess, simply because I am female-bodied, I look around to see who they are talking to. I may be female, but don't look at me when you're searching for the daughter of the Moon. I'm too busy being cranky at trying to get folks to see me as a Child of Father Sun.

Is it weird for a queer sort of woman, like me, who values separate space and time and energy, and acknowledges all sorts of separations as valid, so long as the individuals concede the fact of the separation, to practice what is, essentially, polarity magic? I love women-only spaces, but more than once I've ended up being the masculine element that made them work. Even if the only way I do that is being the butch that carries heavy things, it's a role that I live and work in.

I go to Radical Faerie land in Oregon, and attend rituals there. She's a beautiful piece of land, and I spend so much time being disconnected from the ebbs and flows of nature, living in my urban sprawl, that doing a ritual outside, on land that is lived on and tended, makes me extremely happy. But one of the things about circling with a bunch of Faeries makes clear to me is the fact that this sort of magical balancing is real. If I can be the Horned God, fuck under a full moon at the hole the May Pole goes into, and take care of those parts that I see as masculine, then my brothers in skirts whose magic involves being called "she" don't have to feel odd. I'm the boy with the boys who are girls.

Sometimes my path is that of the servant, and I strive – and fail, since emulating deities can be like that – to emulate Hanuman, the monkey general who serves Ram as the perfect servant. There is dominance in protection and service. There is a path there, when I bow my head and ask how I can serve. There is power in protecting my person, my bottom who trusts me, my little girl. For every spiritual, dominant woman, there is someone who is submitting to her, and that space is just as important. A top without a bottom is a lonely someone with a lot of weird luggage. Someone who can perform the most amazing transformations in ritual is limited, if there is no one to undergo those transformations.

There are ways in which the path is that of Kokopelli and all I want to do, with all my heart and desire, is dance and spin and show off how I can blow my own magic flute. Everyone else should come here and try it, too, on those days. When someone trusts me enough to suck my dick, I feel small and humble and incredibly powerful, all at once. When someone gets on their knees in front of me, opens my pants and acknowledges my strap-on sex toy as my masculine sexual identity, I feel complete.

It's about fucking, which is so often a question of service, really. It's also a question of who, truly, is being dominant. I pack as a sign of sexual and magical competence. I have this thing here, this important part, that will change us both and make us different, and I know how to work it. I fuck and feel changes rolling out from my fist, my dick, my heart into the entire universe. What could be more important, magically or sexually?

Being a masculine kind of magical practitioner is what makes it easier, in some ways, to walk in the day-to-day world as a weirdo. It makes the conflict between being female bodied, masculine-gendered much easier to bear. The important, scary parts of being a guy are solved for me in ritual and magic. I am all the Guy I want to be when I am doing magic, and I don't have to worry about how to do that when I'm in the mundane world. I don't have to explain it, either. It's magic.

Divine Intervention

Raven Kaldera

Monday. Sophia sits cross-legged in her den, silk cloth spread out before her. The phone call she's just answered is from a man who needs her help. He doesn't know how much of her help he needs; he thinks that what he needs is someone to top him, to tie him up, and give him a little fantasy. Sophia knows better.

Before her on the silk cloth is a pack of cards. Not Tarot cards; these were drawn and painted especially for her by a friend. Each has a vision of a Goddess on it, and the cards will tell her who she will be in order to give her friend what he doesn't yet know he needs. She takes a deep breath, shuffles, cuts, and selects the card, turning it over slowly. On it, a majestic woman is enthroned in rich robes of purple and crimson and gold, wearing a crown on her head that is shaped like a walled city. Her throne is flanked by twin lionesses.

Sophia draws in her breath, smiling, and her hand brushes lightly between her legs. Cybele is the Lady she served first, as a galla, the Lady she Sacrificed her past life to on the Day of Blood. With a little chuckle, she remembers how bewildered the surgeon was on her absolute insistence that her Sacrifice be performed on the Sanguinaria, the Day of Blood in March. "I don't do Fridays," he had protested, but Sophia had remained adamant. It would be done in a sterile operating room, not on the steps of the temple of Cybele in full view of the populace as in Roman times, and the altered state would be created by an anesthetic rather than being flogged with whips laced with the pastern bones of sheep. The knives would be sharp and sure, not a pottery shard to cut away manhood and create a vessel for the Goddess, but the date, at least, would not be tampered with. Nor the intent, Sophia had willed.

Cybele, Cybele, Lady of the Lions, Protectress of Cities. I drank from the cymbal, I ate from the drum. The foolish Romans thought that the gallae did what they did to become Attis, Cybele's slain lover, but those who knew, knew better. They did it to become Cybele herself.

He kneels, bound, on the floor. He has been here for almost half an hour and his knees are becoming sore, but he knows better than to lift his gaze from the carpet he kneels on. It is printed with images of lions. Then the click comes, the sound of footsteps – his ears strain to hear, and he is mildly disappointed not to hear high heels – and She brushes through the door in a whirl of purple and crimson. He looks up, just a glance, unable to resist, and a whip of a hundred knotted silk cords slashes him in the face. Recoiling, he hides his face against his knees as best he can while She seats herself.

"You may raise your eyes," She says to him, Her voice low and melodic. No, no high heels, just low sandals that wrap around Her ankles. Her diaphanous robes flow like sunrise-colored waterfalls around Her, spilling from Her high breasts between which gleam a gilded lion's head, and Her long dark hair is held in a ramparted metal crown. "While you are here," She says, "you will address me as Lady. Do you understand?"

He blinks, unsure. This is not in his fantasy. "Not Mistress?" he asks in confusion.

Again the whip, this time across the crotch. He shrieks and almost tries to squirm away across the carpet, but She is out of Her chair and towering over him, six feet of queenly wrath. "I am not your mistress, little man," She says. *"I am your god."* And then he is hauled to his feet by the thick collar around his neck and slammed against the wall.

"Do you know why you are here?" She demands, and he wonders how She can make her voice sound as if it is coming from a regal distance when She's inches away from him. "You are not here," She says, "for your petty little fetishes, feeding your interminable erections. You are here to learn how to worship the essence of woman, and that essence is *Goddess*!"

He is hurled back to the floor in front of Her throne, and She resumes her seat. "Do you understand?" She thunders, and for the first time in a long while, he is really frightened. Not for his life. For his soul, which he is not sure he owns.

"Yes... Lady," he whispers. And then, more truthfully, "No, Lady."

"At least you're honest," She says, Her voice rich with irony. The silk whip is put down, and a heavier one of knotted purple suede finds its way to Her hand. "Unworthy little fool," She says scathingly. "You think that worship is about drooling over someone's toes. You think that the essence of femininity is about cunts and fluff and delicacy, about the willingness to cater to your desires." The whip whistles down through the air. "And I intend to show you just how very wrong you are."

Friday. Her hand hovers over the cards, waiting, as she takes ten long breaths. The woman who is coming to play with her today is not sure she wants to be here. She wants to be challenged, and there was a challenge in Sophia's eye, but her gaze roved nervously over Sophia's six feet of high femme as if not quite able to believe she was admitting to her own desire. This will be very different from the last few clients, Sophia thinks to herself. Dykes rarely come to my temple. How may I serve her, Lady?

The card is turned over to reveal a woman dressed in leather armor, a quarterstaff gripped in her two hands. Her hair is cropped short and she seems to be speaking to the viewer as a flurry of snowflakes fall around her. "Ah," Sophia says to herself, understanding now. "Scatha. She must be unsure of her own strength, then."

Scatha, the teacher of warriors on the sacred isle of Skye, who is also Skadi, icy winter goddess for whom Scotland and Scandinavia are named. Scatha, who is also Skuld, the third of the Fates whose magic is skullduggery, who rides the black nightmare for a steed. "I'd better fetch my armor," Sophia murmurs, "and clear out the back yard."

Looking up from the grass onto which she has just fallen, the woman swears to herself that Sophia is at least ten feet tall. The figure that stands over her wears gleaming steel armor over soft white rabbit furs, a steel helm decorated with a black horsetail, and knee-high sandals studded with spikes. Her black hair falls in two long braids tipped with bone beads. She has just tripped her victim with the quarterstaff in Her hands, tripped her as she came wandering innocently into the yard looking for the domme who had invited her over.

The apparition takes a step back. "Get up," She says in a harsh voice, and the woman hastens to obey. "You don't pay attention," She says. "You need to be more alert. That's the first thing we'll work on."

"Wha-a-" Her guest looks bewildered. Sophia/Scatha feints at her with the quarterstaff and she barely jumps out of the way.

"That's better." The goddess in ice and armor reaches toward a rack on the shed wall, takes down two shinai and tosses one to the stunned woman. "Now. Don't look away from my eyes, no matter what my sword point does. Understand?" She lunges, is barely parried, lunges again and scores on the woman's thigh. Her supplicant yelps and backs away. "Come on!" Sophia/Scatha challenges her. "Do you have the courage, or not?"

Something in the woman's jaw sets, and she lifts her shinai again, settling her feet more firmly on the ground. She swallows hard, and waits for the next attack. The goddess of the isle of Skye smiles grimly, pleased with the change in her. Honing the courage of young warriors is never an easy task. This young one will have to prove her worth with a few bruises and a lot of hard work before she is allowed the privilege of hanging from an ash tree carved with runes.

Sophia denied the Goddess for twenty-eight years before she gave in to Her demands. Her shrink thinks that her visions of the Lady are the sign of an unsteady mind, that she is dangerously close to a psychotic break. Sophia, on the other hand, knows that nothing the Goddess asks of her is even remotely like the horror her life was without Her. Now her body has been sculpted into a worthy vessel, easing the pain of nearly three decades of dysphoria, and she is priestess and instrument of a great purpose, greater than she can see.

"Why, Lady?" she asked the first time she knelt before the Goddess in awe and not denial. "What use would You have for a transsexual dominatrix? How could I possibly do Your work?" And then it had unfolded in her mind, and she understood. The work is a holy one, a work of service underlying the facade of oppression. She could beat the demons of her clients at their own game, becoming them, letting them have her face and form and bringing them through their denial of Her. The Goddess flows through her in many forms: Athena, Artemis, Lilith, the Morrigan, and many other names...

Saturday. The underground chamber is cold and chill, and the slender woman standing naked in the doorway wraps her arms around herself and shivers. Seated on the throne in front of her is a tall figure robed in black, Her face painted like a skull. In one hand She holds a single-tailed whip, and mounted on the wall above the throne are many hooks. The slender woman eyes them and shivers again, knowing, fearing, desiring what is to come. Behind her, in the hallway, guardians of seven gates have stripped her of all her clothing, her jewelry, brought her naked to this room. She looks imploringly at the Queen of the Underworld.

"Greetings, Inanna," says Ereshkigal to the shivering Queen of Heaven. "Welcome to my Realm."

Goddess Be Care Full

Dragon Xcalibur

Goddess, be care full
In the manner of treating your horned god.

He circles you, adamant, taking aim,
Brandishing guns in the breeze;
It is only aiming to please.

Think – in your unimaginable ecstasy renewing,
Think – in your vine-twining tree crotch greening,
Think – in your masturbating web-spin bursting,
Think – in your primordial mud-suck making,

Of the life that it is
Within your power to give:

A steaming mug after a hard day's labour,
A snuggling shoulder into a shaggy armpit,
A blessèd grace of tears when he dismounts.

>   Your fertile bowl
>   Warming his ivory,
>   His metal, his stone,
>   His hand-carved pole,
>
>   His cock your heart opens;
>   Your hole keeps his soul.

And when you send him away –
For you will, and he will go –
Let it be, 'let go to learn,'
Or, 'to quest for the true,'
Or, 'out to play with animals.'
When time is due
Let him see love in your banishing finger,
In your face astern, floating away.

For his memory hopes to feel
Your gravity pull –
Scuttled even in outer darkness – hopes to see
The lamp in the window left lit
For the greybeard skeleton, hopes to find
Himself unknowing under your swollen apron, hopes to hear
Your heart's comfort in darkness booming for joy,
To welcome home and anchor him.

"What is hateful to you, do not do to another. The rest is commentary. Go and learn!" So did a sage sum up his religion to a non-believer.

But still, we ask: What is right? What is just? How do my choices affect others? How do I express my values in the way I live? What does it mean to be safe, sane, and consensual in a world that is none of these?

Ethics touch us where we live. Even the avowedly "unspiritual" must grapple with ethical issues. An SM scene throws light on our shadow sides, the paradox of our desires. If I say no and mean yes, is that a lie? If I wield power over my lover, do I deny my commitment to egalitarian partnerships? What does it mean when I give over responsibility to another person; am I less than I was?

Perhaps there is no one right answer, but we ignore the questions at our peril. Our resolutions, tentative as they may be, bring us closer to each other.

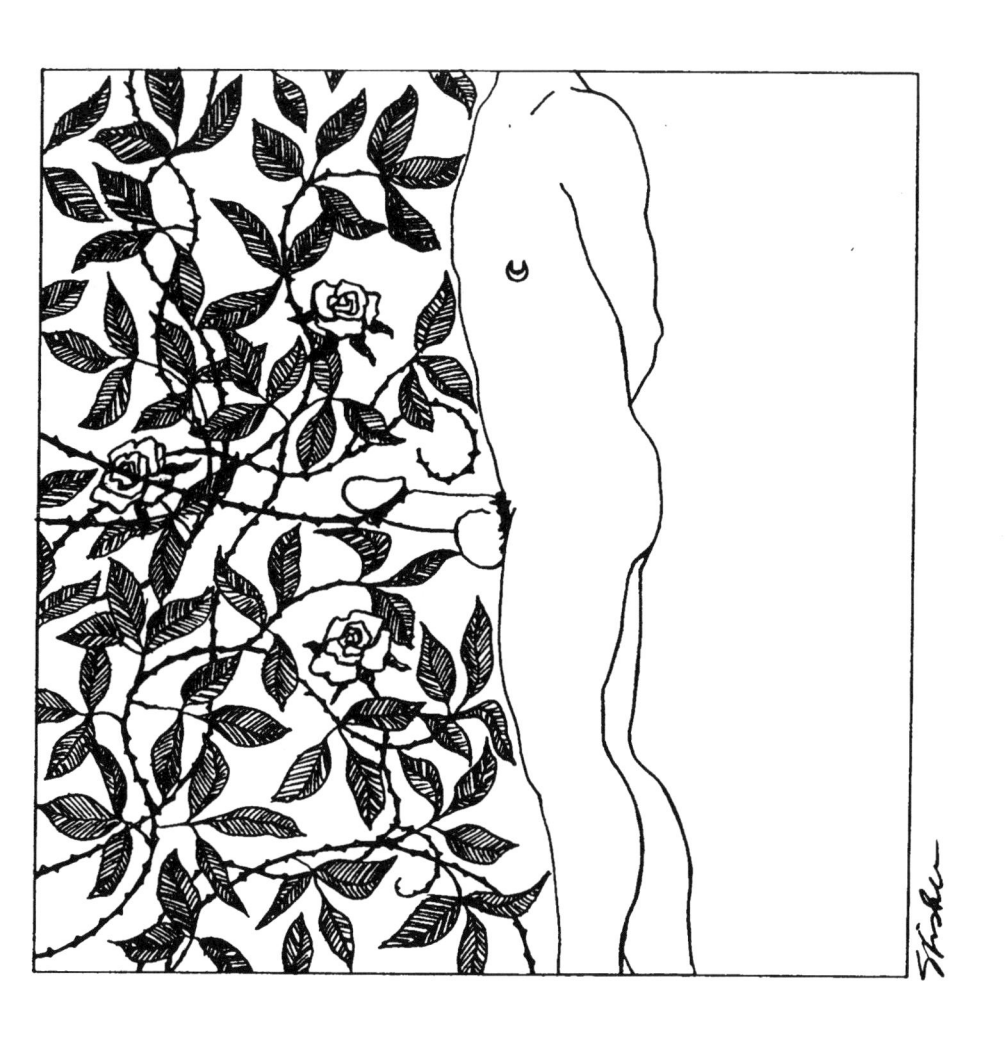

Bitch
Ethics

Toward a Courtly Ethic of Dominance and Submission

Christina Abernathy

It has become fashionable of late to speak of BDSM not merely as an expression of sexuality, but also in terms of an ethical structure, a basis for relationships both erotic and "mundane." By exploring power exchange in a consensual erotic forum, the argument goes, we uncover the myriad power dynamics at work in the rest of our lives as well. Yet this dynamic works equally well in reverse. As more people learn about BDSM and accept it as a responsible and fulfilling sexual option, it is vital that BDSM practitioners examine their own ethical assumptions and articulate them to potential partners and to the larger community in which they move.

BDSM practitioners often pride themselves on their outstanding communication skills, and indeed, the willingness and ability to speak frankly about sexual and emotional matters is woefully rare in this puritanical culture of ours. But when we negotiate, what exactly is it that we try to communicate to our partner? More often than not, negotiation (especially for "casual" scenes) consists of little more than a laundry list of acceptable and unacceptable implements and epithets. While few would deny the importance of this information in clarifying physical and psychological limits, the result is at best, a meager menu of possibilities.

For those who are drawn primarily to dominance and submission (as opposed to physical sadomasochism), negotiation might include a bit more detail: roles, scripting, the parameters of service. Still, for those who desire "deep," transformative submission, these externals can prove inadequate. This is particularly true when satisfying service becomes a spiritual discipline.

In many traditions of both East and West, service is the basis of religious life. Certainly priest and priestesses are, despite their outward appearance of authority, essentially servants of their god and of their spiritual community. Those individuals called to a life of prayer often accept a vow of absolute obedience to their superior. This is the case among Christian monastics who derive their way of life from St. Benedict's Rule and many others.

The goal of service in this context is not glory or fame or riches or any passing satisfaction of our physical or intellectual hungers. The goal is metanoia, conversion of life. By conversion, I do not mean a blinding bolt of light on the road to Damascus – one St. Paul is surely all we need – but the slow, painstaking process by which one's heart and mind are re-formed to reflect more perfectly one's professed beliefs and values.

I propose that dominant/submissive relationships of the long-term variety can provide the stability and commitment necessary to effect such a transformation. I must quickly add this caveat: I am not speaking of occasional "play" or mere erotic titillation. And if one's spiritual path leads primarily to chemically induced trance, what I am suggesting here will prove wholly unsuitable, if not downright dangerous.

I am talking about a move from recreational slavehood to ethically accountable service. In doing so, I am fully aware that the vast majority of people are more interested in simple sexual satisfaction than in talk of spiritual evolution. A blessing on their heads, I say! A sexually fulfilled world must surely be a more peaceful one. But for those few dominants who are familiar with spiritual discipline and are able to view themselves, not as sex goddesses or avenging angels, but as loving teachers and guides, the task of direction may be a gift. For those few submissive souls who yearn to be first and foremost good, mindful, and obedient people, of service to the world as well as to a Mistress, to be a spiritual servant is a worthy goal.

Where do we find models for this sort of relationship? Certainly very few people have the time or inclination to plumb the depths of monastic history. Even if they did, they would find precious little by way of dominant female role models – and after all, they burned Jeanne d'Arc at the stake.

There is one secular movement, though, that grew up alongside medieval Christian monasticism in Western Europe and borrowed at least as much as it contributed to its iconography. That movement is courtly love. Courtly love forms the basis of what can be called the cult of romantic love, the same obsession we see today in its degenerate Hallmark incarnation every February 14th.[1] Courtly love is closely linked to the cult of the Virgin Mary and other devotions that blossomed during this period, such as devotion to the child Jesus and the image of Jesus as Mother.[2]

While scholars differ in their interpretations of the particulars, the basic outlines are clear enough. A young nobleman, often a member of the lesser gentry, conceives a grand passion for a woman of high estate. (The archetypal courtly relationship is female-dominant/male-submissive, although the roles can obviously be adapted for other erotic dyads.) Typically, the lady is inaccessible to the lover, either because she is married or because the difference in their social standing is too great. In many cases, such as that of Tristan and Isolde, Lancelot and Guinevere, or Diarmid and Grainne, the lady is married to the lover's liege lord, making the love doubly forbidden.

The result of this unrequited adoration of the feminine is a great outpouring of creativity on the part of the lover, in poetry, song, or feats of arms. The beloved lady, for her part, comes to symbolize all that is right and noble in the world. She inspires her lover to strive for perfection in the hope that, like Dante's Beatrice, she will one day lead him into Paradise. It is her prerogative to demand innumerable humiliations of her lover and to torture him with slights and deprecations.

Take this example from Lancelot, the Knight of the Cart. In this romance, the twelfth-century French poet Chrétien de Troyes tells the story of a famous knight in service to a famous queen. Lancelot has vowed to do his lady's will without hesitation, thinking not of himself, but only of her wishes. One day, the queen requires Lancelot to climb into a cart – which, the author tells us, was used in those times like a pillory, to display common criminals to public mockery. The proud knight, forgetting his vow, hesitates for the space of two steps, and the queen rebukes him, causing him no end of distress. When the two finally meet again, he asks why she has ignored him, her faithful lover.

Then the queen explains to him: "What? Were you not then ashamed and afraid of the cart? You showed great reluctance to climb in when you hesitated for the space of two steps. That indeed was why I refused either to address you or to look at you." – "May God save me," says Lancelot, "from doing such a wrong a second time; and may God never have mercy on me if you were not absolutely right! [...]."[3]

What kind of a relationship is this, where one partner may ask the other to humiliate himself publicly for her sake? Courtly love, although it is the source of many of our modern notions of romantic love, diverges sharply from its contemporary counterpart in that love is explicitly defined in terms of the lover's service to his lady. The relationship is one of fealty, a vow of devotion to an individual and commitment to serving him or her. Such was a knight's vow to his king, and such is that same knight's vow to his lady love.

What with the unattainable woman and her seemingly random acts of disdain that humiliate her adoring lover, we might just as easily be reading Sacher-Masoch's *Venus In Furs* as a medieval romance! Just as Gregor submits to the humiliation of traveling as Wanda's servant, riding in crowded, smelly coaches with the commoners and sleeping in cold and drafty servant's quarters, Lancelot, the flower of chivalry, submits to the punishment of the cart, the mark of the common, the mean. And all for love.

What are the qualities that a courtly lover wishes to offer his lady? And how can a modern submissive interpret and adapt this seemingly archaic system to his own situation? I hope the following contemporary "readings" of the courtly virtues will help point the way.

I believe that no ongoing committed dominant/submissive relationship can exist without the bonds of mutual affection. Love and acceptance are the basis of such a union. A submissive should be first and foremost a trusted companion to the dominant. Obedience, which often stands firmly at the center of any spoken or written contract between a dominant and a submissive, grows out of the trust established by love.

While friendship and obedience develop between two people, honor is a matter of individual discretion and conscience. Honor is both a personal quality and a system of values according to which we make decisions. It is based on discernment, a realistic sense of order and fairness. There was a time when an honorable woman would not dream of "compromising herself" with pre- or extra-marital sex; a man of honor would not let a slanderous remark against himself or his family go unavenged. For the purposes of a submissive ethic, honor is an internal sense, one which allows the individual to make judgments about a given person, action, or situation. In the most general terms, "being honorable" is an old-fashioned way of saying that an individual has appropriate and consistent boundaries, that he is able to say, "This is acceptable; that, however, is not." It is vital for a submissive to be able to articulate his sense of honor, both in negotiation and in service.

"No, I refuse to speak badly of the Mistress in public."

"No, I cannot serve you in any way that endangers my ability to earn a living or that compromises my physical and emotional safety."

"No, I will not engage in behavior that my Owner has forbidden me, even though I know he'll never find out."

A prerequisite to honor is truthfulness. Truthfulness is the ability to be honest with oneself and with others about one's feelings and motivations and to communicate these as accurately as possible. This quality includes the ability to say, "I don't know how I feel about that yet. Please give me some time to think about it" or "My feelings about that have changed. Here's where I stand now." If a submissive is not truthful, he cannot give informed consent, or more specifically, the dominant cannot be held responsible if, after complying with the submissive's expressed desires, the submissive complains. If he communicates a change in his feelings or perceptions – "I thought I'd like being put in a cage and ignored, but I found out I hated it." – that is one thing. That is being truthful. But complaints such as "You should have known not to call me a swine!" when no such boundary had been communicated are unacceptable. Any sentence that begins with "you should have known" indicates a lack of communication or of truthfulness.

Humility, like modesty, has an undeserved bad reputation. By humility I do not mean rampant self-deprecation. I do mean a realistic perception of one's abilities and desires. This includes the ability to say to oneself and others, "I was wrong," or "I made a mistake," or "I misjudged my ability to do that for you." Likewise, a humble person will accept constructive criticism eagerly, finding in it the nugget of truth that is the key to self-betterment. Often our desire to please is so great that we undertake tasks for which we are not sufficiently prepared. There is nothing dishonorable about striving for a goal; what is dishonorable is the refusal to admit not being able to achieve that goal right now.

Submissives, like knights, need to show **accomplishment** in any number of fields. A lady's maid will need extensive knowledge of make-up techniques and grooming, while a cook may want to attend a culinary school. The most famous courtly lover, Tristan, spoke many languages, played several instruments, was adept at hunting and dressing game, was an excellent fighter and statesman, and played a mean game of chess to boot. Self-betterment in one's chosen arts befits a submissive as well as it does a chivalrous knight.

We sometimes speak with bitterness of the uncommon quality of common **courtesy**. Courtesy is, at base, a matter of respect. If we respect another person's time, personal space, and rights, then we will naturally act in a way that expresses that respect. If we respect their time, we will not arrive late to appointments. If we respect their personal space, we will not scatter our things around their home nor will we touch them without invitation. We will allow them privacy. If we respect their rights, we will allow them to say "no" to us, to maintain their property, and to make decisions regarding their own health and welfare.

One must also be willing to extend such courtesy to oneself. We must, in all humility, respect our own needs for food, rest, privacy, recreation, and the like. It is a discourtesy to others to be discourteous to oneself, in that denying our own human needs makes us all the more likely to disappoint our friend by being incapable or exhausted or otherwise unprepared for service.

Fidelity is a much-neglected virtue among submissives. As a group, submissives are infected with a scarcity mentality, which tells them that there are far too many bottoms and far too few tops. Some feel this gives them permission to speak badly of a former partner in hopes of winning a new one, or to act as if a friend is only a friend as long as he does not stand in the way of a relationship with a desirable dominant. Yet, an honorable submissive can only gain from a refusal to compromise existing, valued friendships.

When a submissive strives to be "good," he is striving after integrity, the sense of security that comes from living in right relation to himself, the dominant, and the world. Integrity implies probity, a view of the self as a rounded and consistent whole.

The essence of goodness, of personal integrity, is compassion, a willingness to look into one's own heart and the hearts of others and be witness to human suffering. A compassionate submissive is one who will look beyond his own good and that of his mistress, to the greater goods of family and community. A slave's acts of kindness reflect upon the dominant as well as upon the slave himself. The willingness to undertake an action simply because it is right marks a submissive as superior; indeed, he may be on the road to perfection.

But what may the dominant hope for in such a relationship? How does she strive toward self-inprovement by directing another's will? I suggest that the dominant must be a living example of the ethics she wishes to impart to her slave. She must always be ahead of the slave in understanding her own motivations and desires. If she is arrogant or petty or deceptive or – worst of all – self-deceiving, she will by her example undermine whatever more formal direction she may give the slave. "Do as I say, not as I do" will not stand up under the scrutiny of an earnest slave; so much less so should it survive a dominant's self-examination.

To ensure the level of stability and patience necessary to train a slave, the dominant must maintain her own spiritual disciplines apart from the relationship, be they meditation, study, ritual, or some form of volunteer service to the larger community. All these lead the individual to a clearer sense of purpose and context. And only by gaining a starkly honest view of her own moral state can the dominant hope to guide her slave to his own best self.

To hold up this model for a dominant/submissive relationship is to move beyond "play" as recreation or entertainment. It demands that the individuals espouse the same ethical ideals both of personhood and of relationships. Rather than gaining unusual skills, like the ability to unlace thigh-high boots with his teeth, the submissive is called upon to grow in moral stature in every area of his life. Likewise, the dominant must display the same level of integrity that she demands of her servant, inspiring with word and deed. It is necessary that both people recognize their own limitations, not just physically or psychologically, but morally, and rather than simply accepting what is, strive to embody what ought to be.

[1] *Denis de Rougemont,* Love in the Western World *(Princeton: Princeton University Press, 1983).*

[2] *Caroline Walker Bynum,* Jesus as Mother: Studies in the Spirituality of the High Middle Ages *(Berkeley: University of California Press, 1982).*

[3] *Chrétien de Troyes,* Arthurian Romances, *trans. D.D.R. Owen (London: Dent, 1987).*

Playing with Paradox: the Ethics of Erotic Dominance and Submission

by Liz Highleyman

Not long ago I told my mother I was working as a professional dominatrix. I had expected her to be upset about the commercial aspect of my work, and was ready with an arsenal of pro-sex work arguments. I was taken aback, however, when her objections were not about the work, but about SM itself, which she believed to be violent and exploitative.

I graduated from elementary school the year Samois was formed. While I had had a few run-ins as a leather-clad punkette with certain feminists in college, by the late 1980s I had found a comfortable home within the leather/SM community. I had heard and read about the "SM wars" at the Barnard conference in 1982[1] and the altercations between SM lesbians and radical feminists in San Francisco, but these seemed like ancient history to me. The debate about the morality of sadomasochism seemed to have little relevance – as far as I was concerned, the "sex wars" were over, and we had won.

Perhaps in no other area of human endeavor has so much ink and thought been expended on ethics and morality than in the realm of sexuality. If sexuality has a competitor, it is surely the realm of power. Thus it might be expected that the ground where these realms intersect would be a hotbed of thinking, discussing, writing, and theorizing about ethical issues. Yet among my pervert acquaintances, the prevailing notion seems to be that SM has attained the status not long ago achieved by homosexuality. It's "just the way we are," and there aren't any moral, ethical, or political arguments to be made about it. However, when I read the writings of radical feminists from the 1980s, I find myself agreeing with their assertion that sexuality is not just a given to be accepted at face value. Sexuality is influenced by societal beliefs and norms – in the lingo of postmodernism, it is "socially constructed" – and that which is constructed can, if we choose, be reconstructed. I believe that sexuality should be given the same consideration we devote to other areas of our lives. "It gets me hot" or "if you don't do it, you can't understand" just don't seem to be sufficient explanations for why I do what I do.

As we approach the 21st. century – with the embers of the "sex wars" largely cooled – perhaps now we can look at the ethics of dominance and submission in a new light.

The Libertarian Perspective

Having suffered the pain of condemnation and exclusion because of their sexual feelings or erotic practices, sexual minorities have often been loath to criticize the sexual behavior of others. Many have therefore adopted the morally relativistic point of view that all types of sexual expression are ethically equivalent. Within this liberal or libertarian framework, it is considered somehow improper to criticize or even question another's preferred mode of sexual or erotic expression. If we want to make the claim that it's wrong for right-wing fundamentalists to condemn homosexuality, for example, isn't it just as wrong to condemn someone for enjoying public sex, being attracted to boys, or inflicting or desiring pain? Within this framework, it's hard to say anything about the ethics of SM besides "to each his or her own."

Critics of libertarian thinking, in contrast, believe that there is a valid place for community norms – and sometimes government intervention – to protect those who are unable to defend themselves. Radical feminists rejected the argument that all forms of sexuality are morally equivalent, and believed that if our sexual desires are "politically incorrect," we should eradicate them and replace them with healthy ones. Within the libertarian ideology, freedom of choice and freedom to pursue pleasure are central values; equality and justice are given less weight. In writing this essay, I've had considerable qualms about even discussing the ethical aspects of dominance and submission, for fear that it will be seen as an intrusion upon people's free choice. Perhaps inevitably, I find myself more often asking questions than giving answers.

Safe, Sane, Consensual

If there can be said to be a community-wide ethic of SM, it is the concept of "safe, sane, consensual." In recent years, this concept has gone beyond an ethical ideal to become a political slogan, even a party line. Yet it is not without controversy. Safety and sanity are not very well defined. It is not uncommon for someone to believe that another person is by definition unsafe if they engage in activities the observer does not approve of. The "false consciousness" argument implies that a person who engages in non-approved activities is not fully in control of her or his mental faculties – or in other words, is not completely sane.

For many members of the SM community (or more accurately, communities), ethics coalesce around the concept of consent. If all participants freely and knowingly agree to take part in an interaction, then outside observers are thought to be in no position to pass judgment on it. While this ideal is widely accepted within the SM community, it has ambiguous standing with the mainstream.

In 1990, several men were arrested in England for engaging in consensual SM. The judges in the Spanner case ruled that consent was not an adequate defense against the infliction of bodily harm. However, they did allow, and most people would agree, that it is legitimate to engage in other activities with a potential for harm, such as elective surgery or boxing. The resistance to injury or harm comes about only when the primary purpose of the activity is erotic gratification.

The words "top" and "bottom" do not transparently describe a consensual SM interaction. It is the bottom's consent that allows the scene to go forward (even in a scene in which the bottom temporarily agrees to forego consent). The bottom controls the foundation upon which the interaction is built, while the top often controls the specific details and direction of the scene. The top's pleasure depends on the bottom's willingness to engage in the interaction. The failure to grasp this paradox underlies many of the moral arguments against erotic dominance and submission.

Some members of the SM community believe that promoting the "safe, sane, consensual" maxim will make SM more acceptable to the mainstream. Yet as with most concepts that have become rigid and reified, other people have begun to openly rebel against "safe, sane, consensual" both as a party line for the community and in their own play. For these practitioners – known as edge players – there are depths of sensation and emotional release that can only be attained if the bottom truly gives up control.

Drawing the Line

While the "live and let live" attitude is common within the SM community, most of us do draw the line somewhere. Most, for example, believe that killing one's partner, even if the partner consents, would be wrong. The majority would say the same about a serious, permanent bodily injury such as cutting off a partner's arm or leg. On the other hand, the majority accepts consensually applied permanent marks such as brandings. An increasingly vocal segment of edge players have challenged "common wisdom" about the advisability of such practices as breath control and blood sports. Given the diversity of views within the various SM communities, it is doubtful that we will ever be able to collectively draw a line separating safe and sane play from dangerous abuse. But we can make a careful examination of ethical principles as they relate to SM in order to inform our individual decisions.

SM and Human Rights

Certain principles of human rights have been more or less universally adopted by societies spanning a range of cultural, religious, and ethical perspectives. Most forms of torture and all forms of slavery are widely considered to be impermissible; some societies also condemn the death penalty. The human rights framework is generally held to apply to states (governments), not to individuals.

Many areas of ethics (for example, medical ethics) give a central importance to the principle of respect for persons. Such respect is generally held to include regard for a person's autonomy and self-determination. Yet within the realm of erotic dominance and submission, how is it possible to honor the autonomy of a person who desires to be submissive, that is, to give up their autonomy? This is one of the central paradoxes of erotic dominance and submission that for many are the crux and the primary appeal of SM.

Perhaps the most contentious issue surrounding SM is that of permanent or semi-permanent slavery. Is it acceptable to regard another person as a slave or a possession if he or she willingly and knowingly consents to be one? Does such consent by definition negate the concept of slavery? Is it even accurate within modern SM relationships to speak of "slavery" rather than imitative role-playing, given that the "slave" can resort to the law and societal censure to remove himself or herself from their "slavery"? Neither the slave nor the master can completely rid themselves of the knowledge that the slave has an out. This is obviously a very different sense of "slavery" than that of, for example, African American slaves in the nineteenth century who had no choice about their situation.

Riane Eisler posits that human societies follow one of two relationship models, dominator relationships, based on fear and force, and partner relationships, based on pleasure, equality, and mutuality.[2] At first glance, relationships of erotic dominance and submission appear to exemplify a dominator model. However – and this is yet another paradox of SM – only persons who are in egalitarian and mutual relationships are able to give the kind of free, non-coerced consent that responsible SM implies.

Hurt and Harm

A crucial point in the ethics of SM hinges on the nature of harm. Common parlance tends to equate "hurt" and "harm," but they are in fact distinct. Having a tooth drilled and filled may indeed *hurt*, but it does not cause *harm* – in fact, it is done to prevent harm. Likewise, whipping and genital torture certainly hurt, and submission and humiliation may cause psychic pain. But are they harmful? I have a working definition of ethical dominance that includes the intention not to cause harm to any participant. Such a definition would include edge players, whose extreme physical and psychological practices are intended to bring the players to a deeper realm of sensation or emotion. While some might dispute their means, their ends are not morally suspect. The definition would not include the namesake of sadism, the Marquis de Sade, who either intended to harm his victims or took his pleasure without caring whether they were harmed or not.

I once had a submissive client who wanted to be kicked in the balls as hard as possible. The woman I was training and I began giving him light kicks, and increased our intensity as he begged for more. It was clear that the harder we kicked, the more sexually excited he became. Since this was a professional encounter with a stranger, we stopped well before the point of damage, but I wonder what I would do in a similar situation in which a lover begged me to bring him or her to greater heights of sexual pleasure by doing something likely to cause lasting harm. In the documentary film *Bloodsisters*, an SM lesbian tells of a situation in which she held a knife to her lover's throat and the other woman said "just go ahead and do it." This illustrates the most profound moment in an SM encounter, when all the paradoxes about consent, harm, submission, and love come together.

While people generally engage in SM for the sake of satisfaction – whether it be an endorphin high, an orgasm, the satisfaction of pushing one's limits, or the pleasure of serving one's top – it is possible that inadvertent harm (both psychological and physical) may indeed occur. Is a practice ethical as long as no harm is *intended* by either party, or is the risk of unintended harm enough to call a practice into question? Certain activities (e.g., suffocation, replaying childhood sexual abuse) are risky enough that some SM players consider it unethical to do them at all. Yet it cannot be denied that some of the most thrilling aspects of life – erotic and otherwise – come from confronting challenges and flirting with danger.

Legitimate and Illegitimate Authority

I have an anarchist/anti-authoritarian perspective, and have sometimes struggled with how to reconcile my political beliefs with my erotic desires. I have been at a loss as to how to respond to questions about the apparent contradiction between my political opposition to hierarchical authority and my desire to engage in erotic dominance and submission. On a "head" level I must grudgingly give credence to such a critique, but on a "heart" level I know that SM can be respectful, egalitarian, pleasurable, and healing.

Perhaps the key to this particular paradox has to do with legitimate versus illegitimate authority. Consent is a big part of the difference between a hot scene and being arrested on the street by a homophobic cop, but it isn't the sole difference. The motivations of the players are also critical. No SM players of my acquaintance engage in erotic dominance and submission with a motive of true malice toward their partner, the way a soldier might regard an enemy civilian or a cop might regard a suspect criminal (or an innocent "faggot" or "whore").

The power of the cop, the soldier, or the prison warden is based not on their personal inner strength, but rather on their role of authority in a social hierarchy, a role granted by a government. To the anarchist, this kind of power is illegitimate. I'm personally somewhat uncomfortable with play that involves police or military roles, because it sometimes seems to glorify state authority. Yet it is just as possible to use such roles within SM play to challenge illegitimate authority. Most SM players believe that such play is a parody of real world authority rather than an imitation of it. Yet critics of SM, such as Sarah Hoagland, claim that "while those parodying authoritarianism may expose it for what it is, they are hardly able to thereby release themselves from it."[3]

SM play involves interpersonal power exchange, which is diametrically opposed to real world authoritarian roles. Such roles are typically unidirectional. One participant is always on top, and the other is always on the bottom. Except in rare circumstances, the victim of the cop, soldier, or warden does not have the opportunity to "exchange" any power whatsoever. Pat Califia has noted that perhaps the reason erotic dominance and submission is so threatening to the established order is because SM roles are so fluid. An SM role is not predetermined on the basis of one's occupation, gender, sexual orientation, race, or class, and each partner may take on the role(s) that meet their individual or collective desires. A top's authority comes from the consent of the bottom (and from the reputation they've developed for responsibility and skill), not from an external authority. Perhaps this helps explain the paradox, noted by Susan Farr, that our society tolerates non-consensual violence such as domestic violence and warfare, but issues strong taboos against the controlled exploration of power by consenting adults. She speculates that perhaps the powers-that-be "wish to withhold experience with and knowledge of power from most people so that abuses of power by elites can be protected."[4]

SM can help people break through usually existing boundaries, such as when a lesbian and a gay man play together. A top in a scene may take on and play with types of power they are never likely to experience in real life. And roles may be reversed – the faggot can handcuff and fuck the cop, the prisoners can lock up and torture the warden. Although partners do not always switch roles within a given scene, and some SM players maintain a more or less constant identity as top or bottom, *the potential* for power exchange is present.

Certainly not all real-world power is granted by the authority of a state. A mother, father, nun, priest, or nurse may also represent illegitimate authority. In fact, they may be even more treacherous because they are expected to be caring and trustworthy. The absolute power that a mother holds over her baby is perhaps the quintessential dominant relationship; at the same time, though, the mother is in a relationship of near complete servitude to the baby. As with state-sanctioned roles, those who play with parental, religious, or medical roles can subvert, pervert, and make overt the erotic subtext of power and authority. Erotic dominance and submission can help us learn about power – how to recognize it, how it works, how to counter it, remake it, and hopefully use it wisely and ethically in the real world.

Dominance and Real-World Oppression

There has been considerable controversy within SM communities about dominant and submissive role-playing that is modeled on racial, religious, sexual orientation, and gender hierarchies in the real world. How does playing out erotic dominance and submission scenarios based on real world oppression affect the ways we either reproduce or rebel against the power dynamics of that world?

An example is the use of Nazi imagery in sexual scenes. Some feel that under no circumstances is it ethical to play sexual games that seem to mimic or glorify ethnic genocide. Others feel that such play may be acceptable in private, but that Nazi paraphernalia and scenes should not be visible in public where nonconsenting people may be present. It may not matter whether a German or a Jew is actually participating in the scene – the symbols and paraphernalia carry their own weight. Still others feel that Nazi scenes have no more to do with real-world oppression than mother/baby or nun/student scenarios.

Ethical issues come into play when people from groups who have traditionally related to one another as oppressor and oppressed play with each other. What does it mean for a white person to erotically dominate a black person or a man to erotically dominate a woman? What if it's a black person dominating a white person or a woman dominating a man? SM critic Robin Morgan has noted the paradox that "he who has power can do what he likes, including playing at powerlessness in a manner never available to the powerless."[5] In keeping with the philosophy of libertarian individualism, many are tempted to say that these interactions are no different from a moral standpoint than any other type of dominant/submissive interaction – after all, "we're all just people." Yet it is impossible to ignore historical and cultural reality. Radical reunionist Hilde Hein has said that "to treat with playfulness and levity a self-chosen condition which is a hated oppression to multitudes of other people is to reduce their suffering to a mockery."[6] In our society, is it possible for people of different races, genders, classes, and sexual orientations to step outside of their traditional places in the social hierarchy and interact as "just people"?

Feminist Perspectives on Dominance

Some of the most heated debates regarding erotic dominance and submission have occurred within feminist communities. Perhaps the opening salvo in the "SM wars" was fired was Ti-Grace Atkison, when she gave a talk entitled "Why I'm Against SM Liberation" at a meeting of the New York SM group The Eulenspiegel Society in 1975.[7] A return shot entitled "Cathexis" was soon delivered by Barbara Ruth-Lipschutz in 1976.[8]

In this era, women were just beginning to speak out about the diversity of female sexuality. Gayle Rubin and others have spoken about how difficult it was to come out as an SM dyke in a time of radical feminist hegemony. By the time I became involved in the debates in the mid-1980s, things had changed considerably. Because of my interest in SM (and my bisexuality), I had never really felt welcome within the lesbian-feminist community, and had instead made my home within a community of perverts. I remember leaving a forum on pornography at the 1988 Socialist Scholars Conference in disgust, striking out with my girlfriend for Christopher Street, where we met some friendly leathermen and purchased sex toys for our later amusement.

The self-identified radical feminists (I find "cultural feminist" a more appropriate term) built an ideology in which female and male natures were diametrically opposed. Men were said to be aggressive, dominating, and death-loving (whether by nature or by nurture), while women were said to be nurturing, submissive, and life-affirming. The cultural feminists opposed pornography, sadomasochism, butch/femme roles, and any other form of sexuality they deemed patriarchal. Lesbian-feminists drew the boundaries of what it meant to be a woman-loving woman ever more narrowly in an attempt to build a safe community insulated from the dangerous, male-dominated world outside their doors. The SM issue was a flashpoint for deep, underlying political differences. The cultural feminists broke with the earlier radical feminist goal of empowering women and giving them more choices in all realms, including sexuality, and found it more urgent to secure safety than to pursue pleasure.

The cultural feminists believed that SM was a male-identified practice. Some, in fact, viewed sex itself as a male realm that woman-identified women could just as well do without. Julia Penelope stated that fantasy was "a phallocentric need from which we are not yet free."[9] Female sexuality was idealized as diffuse and non-genitally focused (ironically, how many people describe their SM experiences), and blessed with a perfect egalitarianism and mutuality. There was certainly no acknowledgment that gender might be anything other than bipolar, or that there could be value in exploring various gender roles.

Most critiques of SM centered around the wrongness of a woman assuming a submissive role; this was decried whether a woman was playing bottom to a man or to a woman. Almost no attention was given to women who erotically dominate men. It was claimed that men rarely desire to be erotically dominated by women (despite the fact that they keep countless professional dominatrices in business). Phyllis Chesler asserted that "few women of any sexual persuasion enjoy sadistic sexual fantasies with men as the masochistic object... only men do – usually homosexual men."[10] Gay male SM was especially vilified as an example of the male eroticization of violence. Andrea Dworkin called it "testimony to the fixedness of the male compulsion to dominate and destroy that is the source of sexual pleasure for men."[11] Robin Morgan saw in lesbian SM "a lesbian copy of a faggot imitation of patriarchal backlash against feminism."[12] SM lesbians asserted that erotic dominance and submission were not equivalent to rape and patriarchal domination of women because SM involved consent. The cultural feminists did not place much stock in the idea of consent, believing that gender-based power imbalances were so entrenched that it was not possible for women to freely give true, informed consent. This argument placed women in the position of children, and did not recognize their status as competent moral agents, thus undermining more than a century of work by feminists to win for women the right to enter into contracts and otherwise be treated as adults. Women's personal experiences with SM were often discounted. Women who had sadomasochistic desires were seen as victims of "false consciousness." If a woman desired to be a bottom, she was thought to have internalized society's demand that women be submissive. If she desired to be a top, she was said to be male-identified. Kathleen Bany went so far as to claim that "to find pleasure in SM is to betray one's female soul."[13]

Bat-Ami Bar On, in what is perhaps the most sophisticated analysis of SM from a cultural feminist point of view, makes explicit that the feminist anti-SM position is based on the premise that "the eroticization of violence or domination and pain or powerlessness necessarily involves a violation of the right to determine what can be done with and to one's body."[14] Yet those who practice SM consent to a rule of masochist control, so that bottoms are in fact in a position of self-determination. Bar On notes that feminist theory does not provide any basis for a response to this paradox. "If sadomasochism is morally evaluated by what it contributes to the lives of those who practice it," she concedes, "sadomasochism must be seen as morally acceptable."[15]

The cultural feminists thought that it was possible to do away with power in the realm of sexuality, and that doing so was the only way women could achieve freedom. Women on the "pro-sex" side countered that power probably could not be eradicated from sexuality, and that we might not want to eradicate it if we could. Alice Echols suggested "We should acknowledge the possibility that power inheres in sexuality... Perhaps we might achieve more equality were we to negotiate rather than deny power."[16] The idea that we can use SM to learn to use power in an ethical way remains, along with consent, the crux of the moral defense of erotic dominance and submission. By exploring the fluidity of power, we challenge patriarchal society's demand that power be "frozen," with one sex always on top and the other always on the bottom.

From the vantage point of the late 1990s, things look very different. The "sex wars" burnt themselves out, in large part because little dialogue was possible and the two sides went their separate ways. There are certainly still unabashedly SM-positive women, but there is less explicit theorizing about SM sexuality. There has been a trend towards an identity politics philosophy in which SM desires (like same-sex desires) are seen as an inherent individual characteristic, not an appropriate subject for public debate. Although there are still pockets of active anti-porn/anti-SM cultural feminism, a more pluralistic philosophy that embraces a wider range of acceptable sexual choices for women has become the norm among feminists.

Ethical Models of Dominance and Submission

Given that much criticism of SM assumes that being submissive is a negative experience, one might well wonder why there seem to be so many more bottoms than tops in SM communities of all sexual orientations. Clearly, many people find exploring polarities of power sexually gratifying. What else might people be getting out of the practice of erotic dominance and submission?

In contrast to the anti-authoritarian and cultural feminist perspectives that eschew dominance and submission in all forms, other paradigms regard dominance and submission as highly moral and responsible. These models often view the dominant as a caretaker, protector, teacher, or provider. If one owns or controls another person, he or she is also responsible for their well-being, much as a parent is responsible for the care and well-being of her child, or a master for his pet. Many SM practitioners have adopted models of dominance and submission that focus on the caretaking aspect of the dominant role. Especially within queer SM communities, the roles of daddy and boy have become ever more common, edging out the Old Guard standard of master and slave. Some women – both heterosexual and lesbian – have adopted the role of Mommy.

The submissive, in turn, is seen as sacrificing his or her own volition in service to another. By subordinating one's will to the will of another, some bottoms are able to achieve intense emotional states not accessible by other means. Submission of one's personal will to the service of a "higher authority" or "greater good" has been seen as a moral imperative in many religions, in certain service professions, and within some conceptions of patriotism and political activism (the nun and the soldier are both models of submission).

People who practice SM speak of many benefits. Many people value erotic dominance and submission for its emphasis on trust. A good SM relationship entails deep trust and extensive communication between the partners. The bottom, of course, must trust that the top will respect her limits and keep her well-being in mind. The top, in turn, must trust that the submissive has a sense of personal integrity and will honestly communicate his needs. Negotiation is an important part of SM play. By explicitly thinking about, discussing, and agreeing to the terms of an interaction, SM players may avoid some of the painful misunderstandings that are common in a society in which sex, romance, and love are supposed to "just happen." Some have found that the explicit practice of ritualized SM allows them to recognize and eradicate the non-consensual "emotional SM" that is a part of so many "vanilla" relationships, for example dishonesty, passive-aggressive behavior, and attempting to get what one wants by devious means.

For many, erotic dominance and submission is a way to explore and challenge personal boundaries and limits; the expansion of old limits and the discovery of new ones in turn contribute to personal growth and the growth of relationships. Some have found that SM allows them to revisit and reprocess past abuse and trauma. By replaying these events in an emotionally and physically safe environment, they are able to assert control (unlike with real-world abuse) and regain a sense of empowerment. Erotic dominance and submission may be healing in other ways as well. For those who were brought up with a great deal of shame around sexuality, being "forced" to engage in sexual play can provide the permission they need to overcome -their guilt. But this is not to minimize the potential danger of playing with painful psychic issues – SM is not a substitute for therapy.

In an era of individualism, in which families and communities no longer have the strength or provide the support they once did, SM play can provide a way to create extremely deep connections with other human beings. It can be a way to dissolve or move beyond the boundaries between oneself and another. Many SM players seek and find a sense of transcendence through pain, humiliation, and deep submission.

SM and Spirituality

Many SM practitioners, as with sexual minorities of all types, have left traditional religions because they seemed to hold little that's applicable to alternative sexuality, or because members of religious hierarchies have actively condemned or persecuted sexual minorities. In my case, as a teenager I left the Catholic Church because its appealing ritual aspects – and its enticing images of pain, dominance and submission – were no match for its negative aspects of authoritarianism, erotophobia, and misogyny.

Within some SM communities, ritual spirituality and erotic dominance and submission are closely integrated. The "modern primitive" subculture, which has grown in popularity throughout the 1980s and is closely linked to SM in some areas, aims to achieve a sense of personal enlightenment and a reclaiming of tribal solidarity through extreme sensation and body modification practices. Most cultural traditions throughout history have included an array of rituals to mark the important events and passages in life, rituals which secular Western society notoriously lacks. Body modification master Fakir Musafar has said. that "SM in this culture is one of the few places people can get started on the road back to their god."[17]

It has become increasingly common within some circles to speak of SM as "sex magick," and indeed, intense sexual experiences can be a direct route to individual or interpersonal transcendence. Some have found ways to use intense pain, physical restraint or immobilization, deep submission, and/or permanent bodily alteration as ritual milestones or rites of passage. Interestingly, people much less often speak of dominance as a way to achieve such transcendence. Roles have been developed within some SM communities to replace the classic SM roles of master/mistress and slave, for example the novice or seeker and the ka-see-ka (spiritual guide). These new roles do not always correlate with traditional notions of top and bottom; for example, a spiritual master might be assisted in achieving a transcendent state through pain given by a submissive piercer.

Others wonder, though, what underlies the search for spiritual transcendence in the realm of SM and sex. Might it be masking an unconscious sense of shame and guilt that makes people feel that SM or sex for its own sake, or for the simple sake of pleasure, is not good enough, and that it should instead be done in the service of some "higher" or "purer" goal? Among queer SM communities, is it in part a response to the overwhelming grief and loss brought about by the AIDS epidemic? Is it, perhaps, an attempt to create a renewed sense of mystique and a new elite as SM has become popularized and its once secret traditions have become available for the asking or the purchasing? Or is it a reaction to the era of the "sex wars" when SM and sexuality were analyzed to death, and erotic desire was expected to be molded and sublimated to serve political ends? If so, it seems worthwhile to keep in mind Pat Califia's reminder that "too much feeling is as bad as too much thinking."[18]

The Dominant Woman

The dominant woman holds a special place in the world of SM. In most of the anti-authoritarian and feminist critiques, she has been completely ignored; if she is mentioned at all, it is as a deluded, male-identified collaborator with the patriarchy. The world views of these critics simply cannot allow for the idea of a responsible, self-determined, erotically dominant woman.

Many of the anti-authoritarian and cultural feminist critiques fall apart when a member of a historically oppressed group takes on a dominant role, especially if they dominate a member of a historically powerful group. For many women, exercising sexual power has allowed them to overcome, at least temporarily, the subordinate social and sexual position of women in this society. This exercise of power in the erotic realm can spill over into other areas, thus challenging societal hierarchies. It is perhaps more questionable whether a man playing a submissive role to a woman in a sexual context will increase his respect for women and his acknowledgment of their equality as people.

While there is no simple correlation between erotic female dominance and women's position in society – we cannot end male supremacy by giving every woman a whip – female dominance does provide a point of departure to explore female roles that don't conform to traditional notions of feminine passivity and submissiveness. Every woman who practices erotic dominance, no matter how temporarily, provides proof that women are not inevitably submissive. While the erotically dominant woman need not be constantly dominant in all facets of her life – and indeed most are not-erotic dominance may provide the taste of power and agency that enables a woman to empower herself in other areas. The woman who practices erotic dominance takes the quest for sexual gratification into her own hands. She doesn't have to cajole or wish that someone else will please her – she can demand to be pleased, or can please herself. As she hones her skills and increases her experience, the dominatrix may become a teacher, assisting other women to develop their skills, self-confidence, and agency as an erotically dominant woman.

There are few cultural images of powerful women, although some do exist in the realms of popular media, politics, and even religion. In many cases, these women do not have a uniquely female role, but have rather taken on a role usually associated with men. The roles usually thought of as dominant within an erotic context or elsewhere – cop, daddy, military leader, businessman, judge – are traditionally male or masculine roles. Common female dominant roles – nurse, mommy, teacher, nun – are not stereotypically dominant, but are rather examples of a stereotypical feminine role run amok, contrasting with the usual expectation of service and nurturing. Women, especially lesbians, sometimes take on traditionally male roles and accoutrements when they are being erotically dominant. Men typically only take on traditionally female roles and appearances when they are being submissive.

Is it even possible for there to be a uniquely female role of power or dominance? Cultural feminists believe it is not, claiming that dominance is inherently male and that dominant women are merely imitating men. It seems that these feminists are reifying women's status as victim by asserting that a woman can't be powerful, and that someone who is powerful can't really be a woman. Yet cultural feminists are not alone in this belief. Even among feminist lesbians who practice SM, it is not uncommon that a top is expected to possess butch or masculine characteristics and appearance, while a bottom is expected to have femme or feminine characteristics.

Within organized gay and lesbian SM circles and the contest circuit, proper dress for lesbians is the same as for gay leathermen (motorcycle or combat boots, chaps, leather vest, motorcycle jacket). The classic dominatrix look (high heeled thigh-high boots, fishnet stockings, leather skirt or bodysuit, cleavage-revealing top) is considered less indicative of power and authority. Must a woman adopt traditionally male signifiers in order to be respected as a dominant, particularly within lesbian and gay male SM communities? Many aspects of the classic dominatrix look are traditionally feminine – and traditionally, looking feminine has meant looking submissive. Certainly revealing clothing, tight corsets, and high heels were not designed to enhance a woman's power, but rather to arouse heterosexual male desire – although many dominant women have succeeded in reclaiming these items as symbols of female sexual power.

The dominatrix role is perhaps unique in that it is not modeled after a real world female role – she is purely an erotic creature who exists solely within the realm of SM. Other roles of female power exist, and are perhaps becoming more common. Examples include the goddess and the Amazon. Goddess mythology has a long and proud tradition in many cultures, but in modern U.S. society, the divine is almost universally assumed to be male. Taking on the role of goddess is another way the dominant woman challenges gender-based assumptions. A small proportion of dominant women participate in organizations that celebrate female supremacy. While it is true that female supremacy challenges the traditional gender hierarchy, it still reifies gender essentialism and the idea that one gender is superior to the other. I prefer to attain and experience my power as an individual woman, not by virtue of the mere fact of being female.

By subverting prescribed gender roles, women who take on a dominant role are striking a blow against sexism. By profoundly challenging accepted societal and cultural boundaries, the dominant woman is providing a positive role model for other women, and contributing to changing women's place in the social order.

Toward an Ethics of Dominance

The most important feature in a community's ethics is not the philosophical framework upon which it is built or the political justification it allows, but rather how its members treat one another. Are we honest, trustworthy, and accountable? Do we interact with consent and without coercion? Do we take responsibility for our actions? Do we recognize and respect the fact that others may have desires and needs that are different from our own? To the Christian maxim of "do unto others as you would have them do unto you," perhaps we could add "as you would have them do unto you if you were in that role." To the Wiccan ethic of "and it harm none, do as you will," we could add the distinction between hurt and harm.

Many traditions, from Christianity to cultural feminism, have positioned ethics and pleasure – specifically sexual pleasure – as mutually exclusive. Yet this need not be the case. We need not give up our quest for pleasure in an effort to be ethical, nor ignore questions of ethics in our quest for sexual pleasure. Ethics is about one's. responsibility to and treatment of others, while pleasure is about gratifying one's own desires. Both are necessary. We can use a consideration of ethics to frame our thinking, explore our limits, and extend our self-knowledge—thus pushing perhaps the most challenging boundary of all.

1. *The ninth "The Scholar and the Feminist" conference was held at Barnard College in New York City on 24 April 1982. Women who were opposed to pornography, prostitution, and sadomasochism demonstrated against the inclusion in the program of certain lesbians who identified as sadomasochists, or butch/femme, or were critics of the antiporn movement. Papers from the conference were published in the anthology* Pleasure and Danger: Exploring Female Sexuality. *Carole S. Vance (editor). Boston: Routledge and Kegan Paul, 1984.*

2. Riane Eisler. Sacred Pleasure: Sex, Myth, and the Politics of the Body. *San Francisco: Harper, 1995.*

3. Sarah Lucia Hoagland. "Sadism, Masochism, and Lesbian-Feminism." *In* Against Sadomasochism: A Radical Feminist Analysis. *ed. Robin Ruth Linden et al. San Francisco: Frog in the Well Press, 1982.*

4. Susan Farr. "The Art of Discipline: Creating Erotic Dramas of Play and Power." *In* Coming to Power. *ed. Samois. Boston: Alyson Publications, 1981, 1987.*

5. Robin Morgan. "The Politics of Sado-Masochistic Fantasies." *In:* Against Sadomasochism, *op. cit.*

6. Hilde Hein. "Sadomasochism and the Liberal Tradition." *In:* Against Sadomasochism, *op. cit.*

7. *Reprinted in:* Against Sadomasochism, *op. cit.*

8. *In* What Color is Your Handkerchief: A Lesbian S/M Sexuality Reader. *ed. Samois. 1979.*

9. *Quoted by Alice Echols in:* Pleasure and Danger, *op. cit.*

10. Phyllis Chesler. "Men and Pornography: Why They Use It." *In* Take Back the Night: Women on Pornography. *ed. Laura Lederer. New York: William Morrow and Co., 1980.*

11. Andrea Dworkin. "Why So-Called Radical Men Love and Need Pornography." *In:* Take Back the Night, *op. cit.*

12. *Quoted in:* Pleasure and Danger, *op. cit.*

13 Kathleen Barry. "On the History of Cultural Sadism." *In:* Against Sadomasochism, *op. cit.*

14 Bat-Ami Bar On. "Feminism and Sadomasochism: Self-Critical Notes." *In:* Against Sadomasochism, *op. cit.*

15 *Ibid.*

16 Alice Echols. "The Taming of the Id: Feminist Sexual Politics, 1968-83." *In:* Pleasure and Danger, *op. cit.*

17 *Quoted in:* Modern Primitives: An Investigation of Contemporary Adornment and Ritual. *V. Vale and Andrea Juno (editors). San Francisco: Re/Search Publications, 1989.*

18 *Pat Califia.* Public Sex: the Culture of Radical Sex. *Pittsburgh, PA: Cleis Press, 1994.*

Death as an Ally in Healing

Reilly

I was at an alternative Thanksgiving party in November of 1994. An acquaintance of mine who was an astrology client, let's call her Acqui for short, was apologizing for being late. She was still obsessed with her ex of six months before, and had conveniently loitered by a park in order to run into her. "What do you think I should do, Reilly?" she asked, turning and gazing at me. She was high, and her continuous whining was frustrating me. I looked into her eyes and said "Stop! Just stop! She's gone. She's not coming back. You have no hope of getting her back. You're being obsessed. Get over it!" She stopped, "You really think that..." I stared at her. "Come on," I chided. She paused, took a breath, "Wow, that's harsh. Thank you." Her gratitude was sincere.

There are all sorts of Bitch Goddesses: those who interfere with domestic tranquillity (Hera, Aphrodite)[1]; those who'd rip your throat out as soon as look at you (Kali, renowned for dancing on top of Her lover)[2]; those who are warriors (Brigid/Athena)[3]; those who are big momma (Demeter/Gaia/Isis)[4]; those who hunt (Artemis)[5]; and then there are those who belong to the Underworld (Hekate/ Ereshkigal).[6] Hekate is the Goddess I incarnate in my healing work.

Carlos Castaneda in his books recounts that don Juan, his teacher, advised him to use Death as his ally. And what a powerful ally. One of the major things in Greek mythology that humans have over the Gods is death. The Gods are often petty. If you live forever you can afford to be. But humans are going to die; therefore we have the opportunity to prioritize our lives.

Now how that looks on a daily level is another story. We all have our issues. We try to hide from them, try to baffle ourselves and others about their apparent shape and origin, but in the end the window dressing has just got to go. Our life is comparatively short and the chance for happiness elusive, especially if we maintain our veils of denial. We all need sustenance, a chance to have our *real* needs met. If we cannot confess to them, the hurdles to their fulfillment become almost insurmountable.

How does this relate to healing? Well, if we all really accepted that we are going to die, we'd be less likely to lie to ourselves that a relationship is working, that the stress we feel on our no-future job is worth the paycheck we draw, that the best use of our lives is to be in constant reaction to the crises of others. In order to heal from her breakup, Acqui had to admit it was over and mourn for the death of her illusions as well as the relationship.

Another friend of mine had ulnar nerve entrapment, much like carpal tunnel, just on the other side of the arm. It took her back going out, and eventually the loss of her gallbladder, for her to leave her unsatisfying data-entry corporate law office job. It was never "that bad." Except that she hated it, and it was wrecking her body. Those closest to her all knew it, even when she wouldn't admit it. We tried to tell her. But sometimes it takes a Bitch Goddess to make you confess your unhappiness and need.

Hekate will do that. She is a Bitch Goddess willing to love you enough to break you into unusual responses. This is not New Age rambling about creating your own opportunity. I have heard New Age gurus blame poverty and the condition of whole countries on the state of their collective "soul." I am no karmic puritan who believes that those who are ill or poor deserve it or have always done something to cause it. That philosophy just strikes me as the victim being blamed once again.

But we forget that we have options. We think we are trapped in either/or: either I have *this* job or I have no job. Many of us imagine either I accept this parent (or lover) or I will receive no nurturing. Hekate, besides being associated with the underworld, is a Goddess of crossroads. Where three roads meet, there is Her place. When we think we only have two choices, both of them unlivable or untenable, we need to remember that all roads have crossroads, even if it looks like a big green field. There is always a third choice that we are either blinded to or has yet to be created. Earth encourages life. Everything has its time, but life is meant to continue.

One of the other ways I relate to the Bitch Goddess is in the style of my healing work. I identify these days as a shamanic top. Clients come to me with physical ailments, emotional issues, or just a lack of connection to deep spirituality. I employ bodywork, herbs, astrology, homework and counseling techniques to aid people in healing and getting on with the rest of their lives.

My work at the moment is not sexually focused, yet many of the joys, privileges and pitfalls are the same as for good SM topping. And like good SM, the work can touch the full spectrum of emotions for both the client and the healer. Frustration tinged with anger has become part of my personal signature.

My anger with certain clients often has several gifts attached to it. One, I don't have to disappear into their need. I can stay clear, centered, and present by showing my true feelings. As a healer, taking care of myself as well as my clients remains a perpetual battle. I feel best about the work when I have responded from my most authentic self.

Two, by my anger, I clearly demonstrate that I care enough to be upset when a client causes herself unnecessary pain. Gushing "Oh, poor baby," can lead the client into feelings of helplessness and condescension. Anger also reminds her that she has a choice – she is not her stuff: Maybe that dream job or lover *is* just around the corner. Contrary to what one would expect, anger empowers both the healer and the healed.

Further, anger creates a sense of authority: I *order* the unconscious to do what it did not know it was capable of accomplishing. For example, a dog can learn how to climb a tree when chased by bigger and meaner dogs. When I order someone to stop, and don't engage with the whirlwind of her self-destructive pattern, it can disable her mental interior voices that are saying it can't be done. To restore self-authority, sometimes it is important to borrow or take the authority offered. It also models healthy and consensual use of power for the client.

The parallel carries further in terms of pitfalls: I heard Pat Califia speak on the "Spiritual Path of the Dominant Woman" at Queer Spirit's first gathering. Although generally familiar with SM, I was new to its intricate workings. I was amazed at the correspondence to my shamanic work. Pat and others present talked about taking responsibility for yourself in play, acknowledging underlying issues, working with threshold, the importance of checking in with yourself and the others present, and reading energy.

She touched on how role and life must remain separate. My clients and I are both responsible for the healing that occurs. We are contracted to be as honest as possible. In my practice, I usually joke about no one dying and leaving me the deity. But I am, in one sense, the deity. So are you and my clients, and rocks and trees. Also, just because I can facilitate someone else's growth, does not mean I have achieved "enlightenment." I am still very much a mortal with my own set of limits and struggles. I "borrow" my power or am a vessel for it, and as such I shape it. But She is the Bitch Goddess, I a temporary means, hopefully to a good end.

I also need to keep owning what are my issues, and not my client's. Counter-transference is an issue for shamans as well as psychotherapists. I need to stay aware of the difference between my personal anger at her (the client), and anger at her blocks. With Acqui, I stopped our astrology relationship and our personal one. While the interaction at Thanksgiving was useful to her, it set the tone for a bad dynamic between us. She would become three or four years old and push me until I reacted and proved to her that she could affect me. I resented those interactions and could not come with full love to them. She was manipulating me to shamanically put her in her place. It's easy for pent-up feelings to linger under healing work. And it's important in healing as well as in good topping to go into a session as clear and present as possible. Otherwise it is an abuse of the power and privilege of the Bitch Goddess.

Yet one of my lessons is the right to be angry with or without a noble cause. Women have been denied the right to get pissed. As I work with this energy in healing, I get more permission to use it in my personal life, and to learn appropriate boundaries with it. Just admitting I'm angry is liberating. The ability to admit what has triggered my anger, to honestly ask for information and negotiate compromise is the icing on the cake.

Another commonality between my shamanic healing practice and SM play is threshold work. I must be willing to love someone enough to hurt them in order to end greater pain. When I trained in deep tissue massage, we were taught that at threshold is where the body learns best. For instance, if I dig into one muscle knot that won't let go, I will dig until there is a cue, such as raising one leg or a cry of pain to indicate this is the client's limit. At that point, I will ask her to breathe into the spot and often the muscle begins to release. If it doesn't, I start somewhere else, try again and constantly search for inspiration.

It's tricky work. The cues can be muscle tension, verbal, breath, or not present. I keep checking with my client to see what the work feels like, is this the most problematic spot, or to find out what feelings come up. I also check back in a week or so, to see how she is, and if she had homework to see how that is going. We may re negotiate homework or how the next session will be structured. In SM, it's called after-care.

Often when I do this work, either physically touching the client or just in conversation, I get images or gut reflexes about what the deeper issues are. My perspective doesn't always match the client's stated malady. If it's appropriate, I tell her my impressions. That way I get further information and the client feels seen and respected. I find great joy in this work: helping someone transform into more of who she is, is profound. But it's also the joy of a top. I give people my advice, even if it's hard.

They sometimes hate me temporarily for it, I ask them if they don't want the advice, and they admit they asked for it. When it goes well, they take the advice, and then they thank me. However, this work is not for everyone or even most. I feel called to what I do in part because of my intention. My main "ulterior motive" is that my client becomes happier and more herself. Even with training and awareness, it's a challenge.

What can you learn from the Bitch Goddess? Well, for a start, let me share an exercise I use to check in with others and myself. If you died, what would your life look like? If you had the chance, how would you live differently? And do those answers change what you need to do now? The Bitch Goddess is clear: She loves you and you're going to die. These are not contradictory statements. Love is not denial. You can hold both: She loves you. You're going to die. The next move is yours. Or it could be Hers. It's your decision. That's a place of incredible power: to really live and to accept that there is enough love for you. The crossroads are in front of you: how about that big green field? Wouldn't daisies between your toes be nice right about now?

[1] *Hera, Zeus' (king of the Greek Gods) wife, was known for causing extreme torment to any of Zeus' mistresses whether they were consenting or not. Aphrodite, the Goddess of love and beauty, didn't much care who She flirted with or slept with, and how much trouble it would cause. She was also known for inducing lust where it would cause the most devastation and indirectly caused a ten-year war.*

[2] *Kali, the Hindu Goddess, has two aspects, one as nice momma, one as the dark mother. She will rip you open and make you confront your issues regardless of whether it will kill you or not. One friend described Her as "Karma accelerated." Volcanoes and earthquakes are very reminiscent of Her energy.*

[3] *Brigid is the Celtic Goddess of smithcraft, sexuality, and poetry. Knives, sex and words of woo – what more need be said. Athena carried full battle gear at all times and was thought to be the Goddess of the Amazons.*

[4] *Demeter is the Greek grain Goddess. When Her daughter was kidnapped, She denied the entire planet food until Persephone was returned. Gaia is the earth Herself, full of floods and earthquakes and natural disasters. Isis, the Egyptian BIG MOMMA God-*

dess, when in disguise as a nurse maid, was granting immortality to a child in Her care, by holding it in the fire. Mom discovered Her and threw a fit. Isis responded by throwing something as well – the child into the fire to be consumed.

5   Artemis, the Greek huntress, was bathing with Her all-woman crew in the woods one day. Acteon, a prince, happened to see Her naked. She turned him into a deer, and his own hunting dogs devoured him. Privacy is so important to a grrrl.

6   Hekate will be described in greater detail later. But I like this quote about Her from The Encyclopedia of Amazons *(Anchor Books, 1991)*: "Goddess of the dark of the moon, and of the underworld, She 'shatters every stubborn thing.'"(p. 113) Ereshkigal is queen of the Sumerian underworld. When Her sister, Inanna, tried to scam Her, She turned Inanna inside out and left Her swinging on a meat hook.

We come full circle. The old/new goddesses stand ready as we prepare to make another turn along the spiral path. Sometimes the path disappears altogether, leaving us to make one desperate leap into the unknown, our own future.

We move through time, our lives reflecting the changing seasons, the inevitable chill of winter. We face our own mortality, our spiritual emptiness, the unanswered questions, the unresolved complexities of our hearts. We pass through a narrow doorway only to find another door before us. Life is what happens as we move toward, through, and beyond these doorways.

Often we are blinded, unaware of the momentous move we are making. Like the Tarot Fool, we step blithely into the abyss. Only when we awake, dazed and unsure of our whereabouts, do we find that we never were really alone. The goddess we cursed as we fell – Bitch! – stands ready to guide us onward.

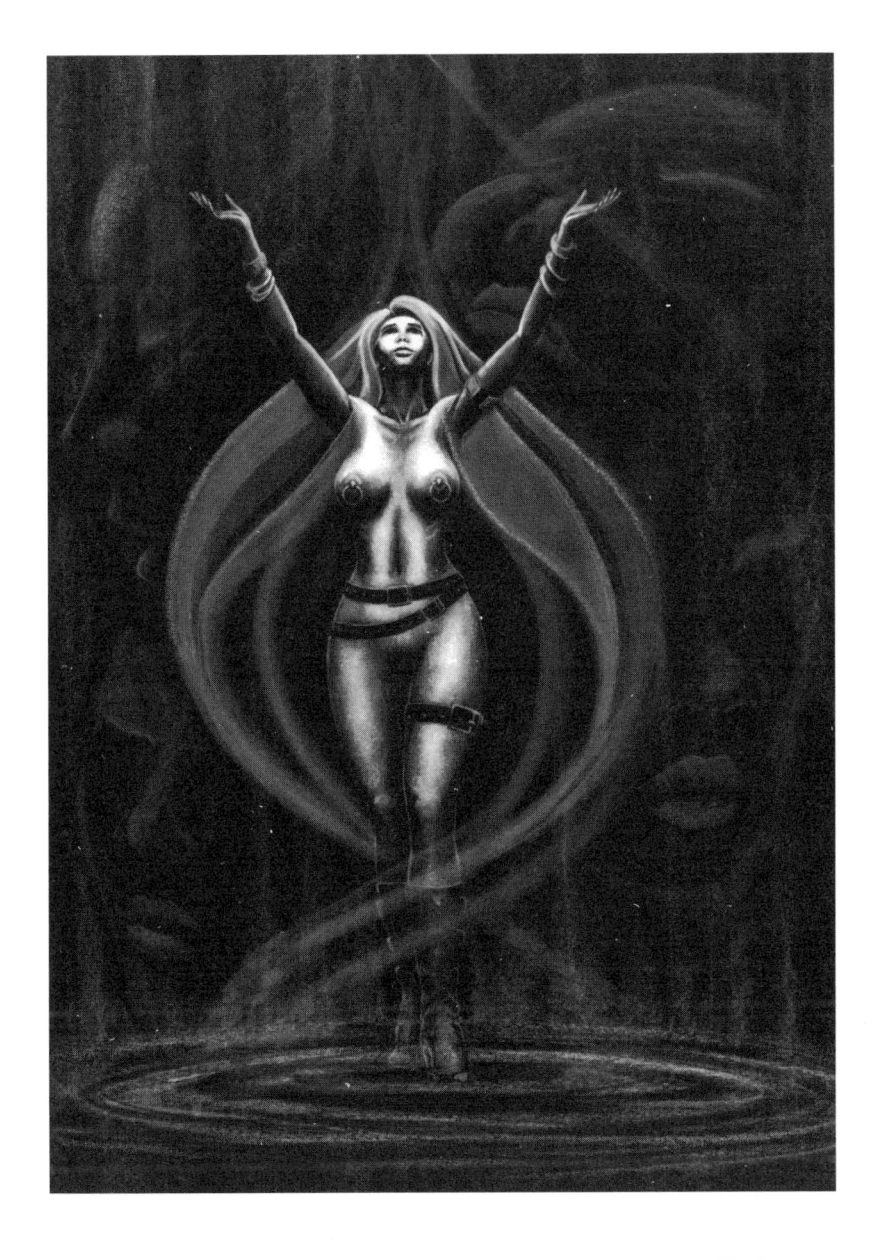

Rites of Passage

Becoming the Crone

Lamar Van Dyke

It was on the chilly side of cold, and there I was sitting in the dyke bar sweating profusely. I must be coming down with some sort of deadly virus. Could it be malaria? Jungle fever? After all, I had spent some time in the tropics. Then it passed as quickly as it had descended. I literally ran home to tell my girlfriend that I'd just had a hot flash. She thought it must be food allergies. After all, I was only 40. I half-heartedly let her talk me out of it, but somewhere in there I knew what was happening. I called my mother. I asked her how old she had been when she did menopause and what that had been like for her. She told me she had been 38, it had been brief, and that at age 80, she still had a flash every once in a while.

I was excited. I never did understand why I had to bleed every month, and endure the ups and downs of PMS. Oh yeah, there was something about it being an ancient curse, a punishment for some old and dusty cosmic infraction. But I had no conscious or unconscious memory of that. I had always wanted to do menopause early and here it was, my wish come true. I was afraid there might be some truth in all the nightmares I'd heard about menopausal women collapsing, with no warning, in heaps of tears; suddenly packing their bags and leaving their families in search of some larger personal meaning in their lives. What about wrinkles, age spots, dry skin, and sagging breasts? And worst of all, I'd heard that my cunt was going to dry up and that sex would become uncomfortable, as well as undesirable.

Oh well, here it was. Another reminder that my existence was, in fact, tied in with something larger than me. I was determined to welcome this inevitable change into my life and just go with it. After all, we all grow older. Our appearance changes. Our ideas and priorities change. I wanted to make this particular change work to my advantage as much as possible. I'd heard about something called post-menopausal zest. I hadn't heard very much about it, but I'd heard it mentioned here and there. I decided to go in search of it, to investigate its existence, and see if it could be incorporated into my life. I'd heard it was the feeling you get when you are released from those regular hormonal ups and downs that we've become accustomed to. I'd heard that when the erratic ups and downs of menopause cease to exist, we are able to maintain an emotional even keel that is so refreshing and invigorating that we have more energy than ever before. I wanted this. I was willing to endure whatever trials would come my way in order to be able to explore this secret hiding place of female personal power.

That was eight years ago. I'm there now and have been for quite a while. It's better than I ever anticipated. I'm no longer a slave to my hormones, and my mind is clearer than ever. I have seemingly unlimited creative energy, and my personal power base feels rather unshakeable at this point. Sometimes I make jokes about getting a face lift. I look at myself in the mirror and see someone who is heavier than I remember her, who is more wrinkled than I remember her... but I also see someone who is pleased with who she grew up to be.

When I was a teenager and very impressionable, a man turned around abruptly, bumped into me, had to look up to find my face and asked incredulously, "What? – are you an amazon or something?" In retrospect I think he meant it as a put-down, but the effect it had on me was immediate. I liked the sound of that word. It made me smile and feel good inside. The only thing I knew about amazons was that they were big strong women who didn't take any shit from anyone and that for some reason they were extinct. They had a reputation for being women who did what they wanted, lived how they wanted, fucked who they wanted and basically determined the parameters of their own existence. It sounded good to me.

After a while I found out that amazons lived in all-female communities. I really liked thinking about that. I'd always felt better in groups of women. It got me high. I ran with a pack of girls all through school. We had lots and lots of fun. When we started doing boys I just didn't understand why things were so weird and jagged with them. It didn't flow like it did with our gang. I matured, I did more investigation, I married one, I divorced him, I married another one, I divorced another one, and yes I married another one and dumped him too. I just couldn't believe that this was all there was. It seemed I needed much more stimulation in my life than what I was getting from men. I ran through them quickly. I had and still have very little patience for boredom and I found them rather boring.

New tribes of amazons were formed in the United States during the '70s and '80s. Dykes hit the road in vehicles looking for each other. We shaved our heads, we ate only organic fruits and vegetables, we worked on alternative ways to do our relationships, and we looked for ways to build new family units. We rejected the patriarchy and searched for new ways to live. We found a power base that nurtured us. We all slept together, we all fought about it, we dealt with our jealousies over and over. We dealt with the fact that we felt like we didn't have very much power in our lives and that life as it was presented to us didn't really have very much to do with us. We began to create community. We validated our hidden amazon desires, rejected everything male, and charged ahead wildly. We started to call God "she." Then it was Goddess. We referred to everything with female pronouns. We took the "men" out of women and started to spell it in weirder and weirder ways.

The Michigan Women's Music Festival began. It was the first time that thousands of women had an opportunity to gather together, with no men around. We got the hang of it really fast. We took off our clothes and lived together tribally for a few days each summer. It is definitely a recognized amazon gathering, the largest of its kind. We drove for days to get there and soak up that energy. We thrived on it. It changed our feelings about ourselves and validated our perceptions.

The less I had to do with the patriarchy, the better I felt. I ended up in Seattle because my van broke down and I just couldn't seem to get it fixed. Here I am 15 years later able to say that everything happens for a reason. Seattle has been good to me and I have been good to it.

Seattle had a very strong lesbian community when I arrived. Lots of dykes. Lots and lots of opinions. It was 1980 and for the life of me I couldn't seem to find any SM dykes. I knew they must be here somewhere, but they were certainly not very out. I put my handcuffs on my leather jacket and hit the streets to find other dykes like me. It went something like this.

I was living in my van in someone's driveway. I was walking towards the street when a woman I had just met approached me, flicked my handcuffs with her finger and said, "What does that mean? Does that mean that you're into SM?"

"Yeah," I said, "as a matter of fact it does."

"Oh, I think that's disgusting. Sick and disgusting."

"Yeah, well we could talk about it sometime, but right now we're standing in the street and I'm on my way out. Bye."

Two days later, this same woman arrived at my van around 11:00 at night. I thought it was a little weird but decided to invite her in to see what was up. She sat on my bed, talking about the weather. She threw herself down with her hands up over her head as if they were tied together. She kept thrashing about striking all these submissive poses while I sat there watching her thinking how bizarre this entire encounter was being. She was still talking about the weather!

And on and on it went. I found the SM dykes hiding in corners doing kinky things with their girlfriends and not talking to each other very much about it. That changed. Seattle dykes came out into leather with a vengeance. We exploded, got wild, had fun and came out, out, out. That history of the Seattle leather dyke community is enough information for a book of its own. But the part of that history that's relevant to this article is that it was a totally female-based coming out. We didn't use the leather boys as role models. We did our own stuff, created our own spaces, and built this community on a creative base of amazon power. Because of that, Seattle leather dykes tend to create wild female-only spaces and events. We seem to be known for that.

Powersurge is one of those events. It's the leather dyke conference that we try to put on every other year. It's a fabulous weekend of gorgeous women doing wild things with each other and revelling in our kinkyness. It's a high time.

Right now, there are a group of women who are working on a cable access television program about the goddess. We are filming women. All kinds of women. We took slides of dyke artwork and projected them onto women's bodies while they were dancing naked to the music of their choice. It's all about how that goddess energy is in all of us and how we choose to manifest it.

My personal power base and access to ancient wisdom allows me the freedom to fly. I feel secure with myself, and find myself ready for new experiences and new transitions. SM, when it's good, provides me with a means of leaving my body for short periods of time. When the energy is right, and the players are right, I enter a space of spontaneity where my ideas and desires take the scene to its edges, not my brain. If my brain is too involved it becomes whacka-whacka-whacka, thank-you-ma'am SM. As a top, I find that boring. I need passion and inspiration to make it worth my while. I want my imagination to connect with theirs. I want them to participate. I don't care if we play with the weed-whacker, or with dental floss. That part doesn't really matter to me. Whatever works in the moment to get us where we want to be is what's important. Ultimately, it's a head trip. It's the high. The toys just help get us out there.

Being a top... I mean, really being a top, is something that has always been inside of me. I am that way. I used to feel very uncomfortable with that part of myself. That was before I found dykes who wanted that from me. When we all started "coming out" into SM, I suddenly had permission to just let that part of myself rip. It was fun. It's still fun. It was very empowering for me to love that part of myself instead of trying to stuff it and act like we were all equal while we powerstruggled over weird things like who was going to drive, or where we were going to eat, or when we were going to leave. It was a relief for me. A big relief.

I'm the kind of top who likes to fly. I like to push myself into areas that I'm not sure about. I like to do new things that may or may not work. I like to take my chances and go places that are, in fact, dangerous. I like to ride that edge.

Quite a few years ago I made a pact with myself that I wasn't going to do any more formula SM. You know, the kind with no passion. The kind where someone I hardly know walks up to me, interrupts what I'm doing, and says, "I'd really like you to beat me." Nothing happens for me. I don't get wet and think, "What a good idea." I just look at them and wonder why they're saying this to me. I want inspiration and participation, not do-me queens.

So now, I'm an older dyke. I know this because I have wrinkles, gravity is taking its toll, and I have more patience than I know what to do with. I feel the same inside my mind. My body is simply going in its own direction. Once you accept that fact, it's sort of fascinating to watch.

I now find that I have a reputation for being a chicken-hawk. I'm not too sure if this is meant as an insult or as a compliment. I'm also not too sure why people find this amusing. I know that I am definitely attracted to high energy, enthusiasm, and spontaneity. I think I would be attracted to that kind of energy and spontaneity wherever I encountered it. Younger dykes just seem to put that out there more often. What this has to do with chickens I really don't know.

If you are used to using lube, which I would think most of us are (after all, fisting without lube is a completely different event than fisting with lube), you don't even notice if your pussy is drying up. Seeing as this was, initially, one of my biggest concerns about menopause, I'm now very amused that I have no idea if this has happened to me. I have lots of good sex in my life, I'm not experiencing any discomfort, and my supposedly old brittle bones are not cracking under the strain of it all.

I was a little concerned about getting involved with someone who is 24 years younger than me. I was wondering if I could keep up... thought there would be some monumental difference in our energy outputs... doesn't seem to be a problem. Thought there would be problems with the difference in our emotional understanding. Doesn't seem to be that way either. If we stay in the moment and the moment is good then it works. If I had nothing else happening in my life, I could probably get involved in telling her how to do hers, but I know that relationships go better if people figure things out for themselves. I have lots of things that are taking up my energy that have to do with me and I find them way more fascinating than things I've already dealt with. I'm very involved with my tattoo business, I make art whenever I have the time, I maintain and participate in my friendships, and I'm discovering that I like to write.

This age thing keeps coming up. It's occurred to me that when I'm 72, she'll be 48, which is the age I am now. I suspect at that point I might be too old for her. I'm doing personal research in this area. I find myself looking at women in their seventies and wondering if I would fuck them. I find myself searching for that elusive spark of sexuality in what we consider to be the geriatric set. Sometimes there's something about their eyes and sometimes I want to touch their skin. I've heard that it's unbelievably soft. But really, it all seems to come down to the cellular memories and experiences that you access when you have sex. It's where you go when you close your eyes, it's how you feel when you pool your energies. Oh yeah, there's the curve of a hip or the line of a jaw. But physical attraction is so dependent on who lives inside of that body. If someone's body is old then you have an opportunity to access their experience, access their knowledge, and of course, access their expertise.

What's the spark that gets you there? How do we cross the line between respecting our elders and fucking their lights out? How do we as older women make it clear that we're still interested in sex, fun, and rock-and-roll? How do we grow old gracefully and stay open to new and unusual experiences? For myself, I find that if I stay in the present it really helps catapult me into new arenas. If I fall into reminiscing about old times, or old fears, then I'm stuck in the past and not able to fully participate in the present. If I get stuck on the negative aspects of the present, then I'm held back by that negativity and unable to experience new and positive aspects of myself. If I start to future trip and freak out about being a bag lady or an abandoned old woman living alone in a room, then it affects my present. I work hard to stay in the present. It makes me feel the best.

Aging comes with tons of negative baggage. It's thrown at us every day. Of course we're going to fear it. But it can go however we want it to go. We simply have to concentrate on having control of our thoughts. Our thoughts determine the reality of our lives. We can have as much or as little sex as we want. We can get involved with women of many ages and learn things about ourselves from all of them. As I become more of a crone, and my friends become more cronelike, I see the power inherent in our aging.

The power of the crone comes from not caring what other people think about us. It comes from caring what we think of ourselves. It comes from basing our criteria on our own experience, not on other people's values and judgments. It's the power of self-confidence and integrity. It's not based on how we look, it's based on who we are and what we care about. I think crones are simply amazons grown older. Women who have accessed our amazon ancestry and who draw their strength from their knowledge and understanding of where we come from. Dykes who don't get sucked into all the bullshit that's out there that's designed to make us feel bad about ourselves.

The Seattle leatherdyke community is very spiritually diverse. There are dykes who observe the pagan high holidays and who like to dance naked around a bonfire. There are dykes who like to incorporate their spirituality into their SM play. Sex-magic can be fun as well as enlightening. However you approach it, playing with power is fun. My personal spirituality is based more on fun than it is on anything mystical. I like to create spaces where we can have fun and get high on that fun together. I'm not trying to prove anything to anyone, I'm just trying to stay true to myself and raise our collective vibration whenever an opportunity presents itself. I'm not the kind of person who meditates, prays, goes to New Age churches, or dances naked around the bonfire. I avoid any kind of organized spiritual approach that is designed to make us think it's all very complicated and difficult to unravel. I think it's really very simple. The secrets of the universe are hiding inside each and every one of us. All the information we need is right here inside of us waiting to be uncovered by our conscious selves.

We can access this information in lots of different ways. SM is one of those ways. When we leave the heavy baggage of our bodies behind and fly through the cosmos, it makes us stronger. It connects us to our roots and gives us confidence to be ourselves. If we do things that scare us, it makes us feel powerful. We overcome our fears and life becomes a little easier.

So we struggle, we fly, we fight, we learn. We've created diverse lesbian communities that support and encourage us to follow our dreams. There's dyke everything. Bars, restaurants, businesses of all sorts. Magazines, books, workshops, and gatherings. This is our community. This is our creation. These things weren't always here. It used to be difficult for us to find each other, but no more.

The young dykes come along now and get to take all of this for granted. I find this exciting because they will be pushing the boundaries even further and blasting whatever constraints they encounter along the way. I want to participate. I don't want to be one of those old dykes who used to do lots of things. I don't want to look like I got stuck in the '70s or '80s, with a tail in my short hair and tight uncomfortable jeans. I want to be here now, learning, growing, and understanding what's happening. I want to keep on moving. I have made a commitment to myself to keep on moving. I intend to honor and enjoy every moment of that commitment.

Empty Me. Fill Me.

By Lady Bachu

The blue-jeaned butch kneels quietly in front of me. I lean forward, feel my painted eyes glow green.

"Show me..." A quiet hiss.

No need to tell her twice. She is well-trained. She steadies herself and unbuttons her shirt, pale blue eyes fixed on mine. One by one she undoes each button. One by one her breasts emerge. A silver hoop on each nipple. A silver bell on each hoop.

They make me smile, these bells. What whim of fancy made her decide to pierce her nipples and string them with sterling silver bells?

"Did it hurt?" I had never asked her before and now I am curious.

She nods yes.

"What happened?"

She closes her eyes, silent for a moment. "I screamed at the first one," she admits.

I clearly saw the moment of piercing and my flesh itched. Those silver bells hold a certain fascination for me. But they also leave a bitter taste of revulsion on my tongue. I reach out my finger and tap the shiny ornament decorating her right nipple. Instantly an echo of her scream rings through my inner ear. The shriek. The moan.

I feel sick. This is not good. This woman comes to me, offering herself over and over to me. "Empty me, fill me," she says. "It doesn't matter."

Empty me. Fill me. Empty me. Fill me.

Sadness rises from the center of my belly and closes my throat. This is a soft sadness, soft as new snow falling from a sodden sky.

I swallow my sudden pain and sadness. "Come with me, " I tell her. I rise. She follows. She always follows. I love counting on her for that. I lead her into the bathroom. Turn on the tub faucet. Let it begin to fill.

I turn to her again, bare breasted except for those tiny bells. She waits. I pull her toward me and cover her mouth with mine and begin to kiss her slowly. I empty her with my kiss, draw breath from her, fire from her, obedience from her, devotion from her. Empty me. Fill me. I take all from her with that kiss. Feel her drop as she gives it all up. And still I keep kissing her. Kissing her and taking every fear, every hope, every laugh, every shriek that has ever roosted in her bony frame.

And when I am done kissing her dry, I gather her up boots, bells and all, and place her in the warm tub of water. Ready to begin the filling again.

For B.

Catherine A. Liszt

I strain to hurl the whip
as though its fingers could pass right through her
combing every cell in her flesh
into orderly lines
pointing due north
quivering and constant

I am not that strong.

So I make her scream
knowing that sound echoes forever
and hoping that in some frightened future
a note of her music
will come into my ear
and say welcome

Such a lonely hope.

I reach up inside her
and feel my bones grind together
trying to find the spark
so I can cup my hand around it
and shelter it from a wind
too powerful for any protecting.

Breathe, my love, breathe.

Goddess

James Williams

I remember the colors your living room featured long after dinner the April evening when we met. You lounged in the deep blue sofa facing the fireplace; I waited on the edge of a soft rose chair beside you. The yellow candles had long since guttered and our amber brandies glinted in the fight of the logs' orange embers. A waning moon the color of butter presaged dawn beyond the windows at my back and lit the bones and hollows of your face so boldly I could almost feel your flesh.

All your other guests had gone and I had begun to feel awkward, since there was obviously no excuse for me to stay. Yet I could not bring myself to stand and mouth the usual platitudes of thanks and farewell. From the moment I had seen you I had been drawn to you – to your beauty, of course, but even more to your vibrancy, your intelligence, your playfulness, and most of all to your emotional *presence*, which I felt encouraged me to be intimate with you: to know you, and allow you to know me.

More than once I took my eyes from yours because I wanted to stop the longing I felt welling up in me; wanted to stop the longing before it became too visible; before I spoke inappropriately and said something you might not want to hear; before, in a sense, I exposed myself to you without permission. But every time I took them away I brought my eyes back to yours, because more than I wanted to stop my feelings I wanted you to feel them too: to feel the corresponding desire growing in your breast, swelling your lips and moistening your thighs; I longed for you to *want* from me what I wanted so greatly for you to take.

You still wore the plain, black, high-necked leather jerkin one guest had said made you look like an ancient deity, and on this soft skin, below your throat, a long, clear crystal pendant rested. As I stayed a minute and a minute more your fingers lit upon that pendant and lifted it up, and with an eye cocked my way you drew its narrow tip along your lips. Black curls tumbled down your tilted head and framed your eyes in a bandit's mask. Your sidelong look became a gaze that entranced me. I felt I could not escape from you, nor did I think I would ever want to.

Only the language of love as divine has devised words for the feeling I had, so the more completely I recall the night, the closer I come to the breath of passion: to saying I wanted to give you my life, to feel your teeth break my boundary of skin and your mouth suck out my very soul and make my spirit spill.

I must have spoken then because, although I felt confused, I wasn't surprised that you replied. "Goddess?" you asked. "Did you call me 'Goddess'?"

Had I? I didn't know, and you seemed to find in my dilemma a source of genuine merriment. Your voice was as clear, your laughter as musical as glass bells. "I like to be seen for the Goddess I am," you said, cautioning me with the crystal finger, "but I am a Goddess who makes demands, not one who necessarily grants favors. Are you ready to worship, and serve, and supplicate? Is that what you have in mind?"

I stared at your dark eyes, and the mischievous smile in your lovely human face. I fell into whatever the play was that I seemed to have begun myself. "Yes, Goddess," I replied, "I am ready for that; that is exactly what I have in mind."

You leaned on one elbow with your chin in your hand and looked me over as if we'd never met before; then "Down," you said, pointing to the floor before you. I came off the chair and dropped to my knees in a single movement, torn between my urge to prostrate myself before you and my equally strong desire to remain on my knees looking into your eyes so I could see the heat of erotic power rising up in you. Showing the tiny pink tip of your tongue, you sat up on the couch and raised one booted foot to rest upon my shoulder. I wanted to bury my face in the flesh you bared, startling white beneath your black skirt, but you let the weight of your foot impose, and I bowed my neck to your command.

I pressed my lips to the top of your other boot as the pressure of your foot demanded, kissing in the valley between your toes and the bone that rose above the arch. I did not aim my kiss at the supple leather my mouth met but at your foot beneath it, which was part of you. I sought to let you feel how deeply I wanted to submit my will to yours, to serve your desires, to follow you to the edge of my self until I lost all sense of me and begged you to let me vanish into you. My body shook for the first few times that night and I felt the tears of my first small passionate release. You removed your foot from my neck. "Up," you said. I rose on my knees and spread my arms to you.

"Thank you, thank you, yes oh yes oh please," I prayed, all but certain you could hear my thoughts, willing my hopes across the wordless air that tingled now like hot slapped skin. You gazed at me intensely, as if envisioning my surrender. You pushed the toe of your boot into my crotch, pushing my legs apart. I was hard and you pressed on my erection. My body responded, pressing back, and you kicked me from beneath, lightly but with no mistake. I stopped for a moment, imagining I was sobered, and took this first pain you had ever given me as if it were a gift and a promise. You nodded once. "That's right."

You leaned back and crossed your legs. I could see the curve of your calf within your boot, the angle of your hip, the small swell of your breast, the waves and curls of flesh that made your mouth. "You may proceed," you said, gesturing at my jacket, "but do not stand up."

As quickly as I could from my position on the floor I undressed, folding my clothes and piling them beneath the chair I'd sat in. When I was naked and kneeling quietly once more you turned me toward the silvery window to give yourself a better view of what was being offered. You smiled at me kindly and stroked my hair, stroked my cheek. I could smell the different parts of you. Erotic tension charged me with desire. My penis swelled and ebbed, swelled and ebbed like a live thing breathing on its own. The air around you seemed to glow. I closed my eyes and nuzzled your palm feeling elated, feeling devoted, restraining my need to kiss and lick and suck and bite and take your hand your arm your body self into me my mouth was dry when you slapped me across the face. My eyes jerked open and I awakened to the shame of my lost control.

"You kiss on command, not on your own initiative." You raised your brows, asking if I understood.

"Yes, Ma'am. I –"

"Do you wish to speak?"

"Please, Ma'am."

"Do you wish to apologize?"

"Yes, Ma'am."

"Don't."

You moved your hands across my chest, tugging a little at the hairs now and then, and let one come to rest massaging my breast. You began to pinch me between your nails: alerting my flesh and taking my attention where you wanted it to go. You pinched harder. I breathed more deeply, feeling cut, till suddenly you let me go, let the blood rush back, and slapped my breast. You held the hand that had hurt me to my lips until I kissed it. "Good boy," you smiled.

Your hands began their wanderings again, over my sides and belly and hips and ass. You came to my cock, which was wet and partly hard, and ran your nails along the shaft. I thought by the tension in your jaw that you resisted some desire in yourself to scratch long reminders of your passing in my blood. You slid your hand down, wrapped one finger and thumb around the neck of my scrotum, and slowly started to tighten your grip on my balls. My breathing quickened and my eyes widened; you grinned and squeezed me harder.

"You like this," you mused. I tried to answer but the truth was so extremely Yes and No, and the pressure was taking me down so far and so fast, I only gasped and stammered. The pain itself was a doorway I did not want to go through, but I knew that it would let me give myself up and make of myself a gift to you, and I did want that. You kept your eyes on mine as I began to whimper, making sounds I did not mean to make. You reached up through me and sought my heart, sought to carry us both deeper. I wanted you to have it; I wanted you to feel that you could own me. I forced my breathing down, and down, slowing the rush of sensations, enriching my response to you.

"Turn around," you ordered. Panting and aching all the way up my abdomen, light-headed and in awe to feel controlled by my balls in your surprisingly strong hand that neither softened nor let go, I managed the awkward move and straddled your arm.

"Bend over and put your face on the floor. Spread your cheeks. Use your hands. Push out. Pull in. Push out. Pull in. Again. Again." You slapped my cheeks beside my hands, first on one side then the other, lightly at first then harder and harder. Abruptly you slapped directly on the tender inner skin I'd opened for you. I tightened up, and when I relaxed you slapped again and again, stinging me repeatedly until I stopped fleeing and eased myself onto the gentle probing of your finger. You came inside me, moved around, moved in and out, probed some more, pressed and pulled and opened me farther. Pushing up against me with one hand and bearing down with the other, suddenly you broke through me. I cried out, let go, fell sobbing on your arm and pushed myself deeper into your tightly balled fist, relieved to live as if forever beneath your will, taken, surrendered, turned over, possessed, your human property at last; you let go and I screamed as the pain of release rose snaking to my brain.

"Now," you murmured, listening to me cry, "now we can begin."

Slowly you withdrew your hands from me. I shook as I wept before you and wept for you on the floor. I reached devoutly for your feet but you just pulled away. "Ask," you said. "No: *beg*."

Joyful, despairing, proud to give this up to you, I started to obey but lost myself in the meaning behind my words. "Oh Goddess, Goddess," I began, "please please please please please may I hold you, please may I hold your legs, please may I kiss you, please may I..." please may I please you, please may I live for you, please may I die for you, please will you use me, abuse me, hurt me, humble me, amuse yourself with me, take me beyond myself, let me stay with you, let me live in you, let me disappear upon your hands and hold this holy moment in your eyes with mine –

"Yes, you may."

I grasped your legs and pressed myself as far as I could to merge with you from the floor. As my shuddering subsided and peace took me over you prodded me onto my back and rested your feet on me. Through my fading psychic haze of pain I heard you move in your seat; later you shook me with a foot against my face. "Time to serve, my pet. Kneel up."

*

"There are some things to do before we get fully started," you said. You sent me scuttling to a chest beside your desk, and had me bring back a zippered bag you opened slowly, watching me watch your hands. You took out a plain black collar with a D-ring opposite the buckle and put it to my lips to kiss. I agreed – eagerly, gratefully – to be your slave until you took it off: to obey and serve you as you commanded me to do, to honor and worship you in the ways you directed, to accept without question whatever punishments and rewards you might mete out.

After I agreed you told me to bow my head, and when I felt you wrap your collar around my neck all the tension of the night drained from my body and I felt free. You buckled and locked the collar in place and lifted my chin; I looked up at you with a growing sense of veneration. You brought out a much smaller collar with a smaller D-ring and had me kiss that as well. One side of your mouth turned up as you wrapped it around my scrotum where your finger and thumb had captured me, and snapped its lock shut as well. The little metal sound reverberated in my skull like the echo of a heavy prison door banging closed. You took out a chain with a black leather handle and clipped it to the collar at my neck. How happy I was, how near to ecstasy, on my knees, in your collars, and in your thrall.

"Down," you said, "on your hands and knees. When I say 'heel' you are to follow me. Stay out from under my feet so I don't have to trip over you, and pay attention to the leash so that you stop when I do, without my having to speak to you. Do you understand?"

"Yes, Goddess," I replied.

"Good. Then 'heel'."

Every movement I made took me farther out of the deep place I had been, yet each was also a sign of my obedience, and a step along the road of my submission to you. You stood and walked me up and down your living room, turning figure eights until I stumbled; then you shortened the leash to hold my face against your knee. I followed you through the hallways of your house from room to room, keeping my eyes on your moving feet, dancing backwards and to the sides, learning to match your rhythm as you changed speed and directions. When you stopped we were on the cool apricot tiles of your bathroom floor. "Not bad," you said as you sat in a wicker chaise against a mirrored wall and draped the leash my shoulders; I caught my breath and presented myself before you. "Draw me a bath, warm, not hot."

I plugged the tub and turned the water on, testing it with my hand as the pastel basin filled.

"Undress me, starting at the top. Do not remove my pendant."

When you signaled that you were ready I removed your clothing piece by piece, and as I exposed your body I worshipped it in my heart, shoulder to back to arm to breast to belly to cheeks to lips to legs and feet. At first you held yourself a bit apart from me, testing the bounds of this physical intimacy, testing the trust we were building between us, but I did not touch you more than necessary to unbutton and undrape because you had not yet been pleased to tell me to touch you anywhere at all.

You sat in your bath, closed your eyes, and sighed, luxuriating in the water's warmth while I knelt beside the tub. After awhile you said, "My sponge is on the shelf behind me. Use the lilac gel. Do my face first, only with your hands, then use the sponge starting at my shoulders and work your way down to my feet."

I set the sponge in the bath to soften while I coated my hands with gel, and as I gently bathed your face, kissing it with my fingertips, I watched your jaw relax, and your eyelids relax, and some of your life's cares ease. After I rinsed your face I filled the sponge with gel and bathed your shoulders, your arms, your back, your breasts.

You stood in the tub for me to wash your belly and – gradually, leaving you plenty of time to stop me if I was wrong – your pubic mound and vulva; then you turned around so I could wash your buttocks and, delicately as you bent forward, your anus. You sat again to cover yourself with water, and let me lift first one leg then the other so I could sponge each one from thigh to toe.

"Another time I'll teach you to wash my hair," you said as you stepped from the tub and wrapped yourself in the towel I handed up to you. "For now, I think, you can simply – soak in my bath."

You unclipped the leash and set it on the chaise. You snapped your fingers and I almost leapt into the pale gray water that was still warm and smelled of you and lilac soap. "Down. All the way down. Put your face in it." You placed your foot on my head and held me under water for a few long seconds, then let me up to breathe again. "Now I am on your outside," you said. "I want to be inside you as well." You stepped into the tub again, positioning yourself immediately above me. You gripped my hair and tilted my head back.

"Open wide." When I opened my mouth you started to let your urine flow, first a little dribble down your leg, then a full stream flushing my face. Using my hair as a hand-hold you pulled my mouth to you. "Swallow," you commanded. "Drink it all."

I didn't know I had anything more to give you but I reached and did as I was told. When you were through I was gasping for air. The smell of you filled my nose and the taste of you filled me from my stomach to my lips. I saw your eyes, amused and satisfied. I wanted to weep when you smiled at me. You pulled my head forward and let me lick you clean in silence, stepped from the tub and pointed at the floor again. I clambered out and knelt beside you. You dropped your towel on me and told me to rinse my face and dry myself. You filled a glass with water and handed it to me.

"Wash your mouth out," you said. "Even a Goddess's piss is acid. It's not good for your teeth."

After I had rinsed my face and mouth and swallowed the water as you told me to do, you reattached the leash to my wet collar. "Heel."

You walked me to your bedroom and took a large clean sheet from a dresser drawer. You handed me the sheet and showed me a tray of unguents. You told me to spread the sheet over the bed, and said you wanted a massage. You said I could stand and walk around as necessary in order to perform these tasks. You looped the leash around my neck, put on some simple music whose soft rhythms made the room seem like a temple, and after I had stood and covered the bed with the sheet you lay face down upon it.

I stretched my own tired limbs and consulted the tray full of bottles. I selected a delicately scented floral lotion, poured some into my hand and put the bottle down, then warmed the lotion between my palms. Finally I touched your neck and shoulders and gradually rubbed lotion down into your back and buttocks and the backs of your legs. I soothed your flesh from your thighs down toward your ankles, smoothed the tight webs of muscle from the heel forward, pressed lotion into your feet through the outsteps and around the balls, through the insteps and under the toes, spread the bones and stretched the ligaments, opening your soles to the earth. Finally I brought your feet together, wiped them down with the towel, and wiped my hands.

I stood beside the bed and waited. Across the room your mirror reflected back to me the image of a middle-aged man in respectful service: naked and open, idle hands held out of the way behind his back, collared at the neck and genitals with a leash draping off one shoulder down his chest, owned and available for – for you. Feeling myself under a Goddess's control filled me with joy and made me want to laugh. Beside my image in your mirror I could see your image stir. You rolled over onto your back and said, "Continue."

Again I started with warm lotion at your chest and shoulders where your pendant glittered on its chain like ice. I smoothed the lotion up along your throat and down your ribs, stretching your arms, pulling and pressing on your breasts and yielding belly, working toward your feet. When I was done I stood at your head and wiped your brow, and spread stray wisps of hair off your face. After a few minutes you opened your eyes and stretched. "In the kitchen, in the refrigerator, you will find an open bottle of wine," you said. "Beside the refrigerator you will find a crystal goblet. Fill the goblet with wine and bring it to me."

I went off to do as I was told. When I returned I knelt and proffered the goblet as if it were a sacrament. You took the goblet from my hands and set it down beside you, then held my face with one hand and slapped me smartly with the other.

"Who told you to?" you demanded.

"Goddess?" I cried, stung.

You slapped me again. "Who told you you could walk when you went to fetch my wine?"

My heart fell. "No one, Goddess."

"Do you decide these things for yourself?"

"No, Goddess."

"Why did you?"

"I made a mistake, Goddess, and I am deeply sorry."

"As well you might be. You shall be punished later. Do you understand?"

"Yes, Goddess."

"Good. Then you may entertain me now. Stand up – " I stood " – and do some jumping jacks."

"Excuse me, Goddess?"

"Jumping jacks. You don't know what those are? You jump in place, and as you do so you spread your legs and clap your hands over your head. Then you jump again and bring your legs together and clap your hands to your sides. That's a jumping jack. Then you repeat the movement until I say to stop. Do some jumping jacks for me."

Feeling foolish and older than I wanted to be I started doing jumping jacks. Each time I jumped my genitals bounced up and down. Leaning against the headboard of your bed sipping your wine, you began to smile.

"Stop," you said, and I stopped. "Down," and I knelt. "Come," and I crawled to you. You released the leash from the collar at my neck and reattached it to the collar at my balls. "Stand," you said. "Jump." You gradually shortened the leash until each time I jumped the collar tightened, making me my own tormentor.

"You're slowing down," you said, slapping at my flopping cock with a riding crop you'd taken from your bedside table. "Don't do that. Jump. Jump higher."

The doorbell rang and I thought I might be saved, but you had another plan. "Stop." You attached the leash to the collar at my neck again, and hung the leash around my neck. "Jump." I started jumping. "Keep jumping until I return." And with that you left, trailing the scent of the lotion I'd massaged you with, that smelled like the last spring flowers in the first summer rain.

I was tired and sweating, my thighs and calves were quivering from exertion, my knees were sore from kneeling and crawling, my balls hurt from being squeezed and pulled, my cock hurt where you had cropped me, my mouth and breath tasted of your urine, and I hadn't pissed in hours. Left all by myself with this inane instruction to jump until who knew when I thought that maybe I had come to the wrong place, was doing the wrong thing, was playing the wrong game. Why did I want so deeply to please a woman I had never met before? Why didn't I just want to please myself? What kind of idiot was I, anyway? Why didn't I at least just cool it till I could hear you returning? Then I could resume this jumping – you'd never know the difference.

But I saw myself in the mirror again, and instead of seeing the tired man, I saw again the collars that belonged to you and with which you had claimed me, and I knew I couldn't fake it: I knew if you were really able to hold me, I had to let myself be held by you. Sighing then, I jumped, and I jumped, and I jumped.

After only a few minutes you returned, wearing a loose robe and accompanied by another woman who cast a brief glance at me, then turned her attention to the tray of lotions, oils, and powders.

"Stop," you said. You pointed to the floor beside you and I knelt on the spot, breathing hard.

"Are you tired?"

"Yes, Goddess," I replied.

"You may rest." You pointed to your feet, where I lay my forehead. I felt so grateful for this little respite I wanted to cry.

"Do you need to drink?"

"Yes, Goddess."

"Do you need to urinate?"

"Yes, Goddess."

"Come. Heel."

On hands and knees I followed the leash as you led me from the bedroom, down the hall and over the white living room carpet, past the blue couch and the rose chair, past the cold fireplace, past memories of last night's dinner party, and through a sliding glass door into your back yard and the full daylight of a late spring morning. In a far corner, upon a patch of bare earth, lay a rusty trowel.

"This is where you may relieve yourself," you said, pointing to the spot. "Dig a deeper, wider hole than you plan to use, and after you're through fill it up with dirt."

I dug the hole, then realized I had never tried to piss while kneeling – or while a woman held my balls on a leash. Time passed.

"Come on," you said. "You're going to have to get over it or you'll burst your bladder."

Just as I felt myself about to let go you squatted down and grinned and took my cock in your hand. I began to get a little hard. More time passed and now you seemed infinitely patient, enjoying the sun and my discomfort. Your friend came out of the house and the two of you chatted. You gave the handle of the leash to her and she played with the chain, pulling me back and forth and jiggling me around. She laughed, not unkindly, and you laughed with her. I tried to tune the two of you out. Finally I pissed, my urine frothing and disappearing in the hole I'd dug.

"It feels so funny," you said to your friend as you shook the last drops from my penis for me, and then stood up. "The whole thing sort of vibrates. It must be odd to have your genitals hanging out in the wind like that." You and she continued to talk while I shoveled dirt in the hole, then you led me to a garden hose. You put the leash around my shoulders and turned the water on. You let me drink, and when I had had enough you hosed me down all over. The water was cold, and when I gasped you laughed.

You led me to a bush with long, smooth, flexible branches, and snapped a thick one off. You whipped it through the air and it whistled its greeting. You stripped the branch of leaves and touched it to my flank. "Do you remember why I am going to punish you?"

"Yes, Goddess."

"Why?"

"For walking without permission, Goddess."

"Will you disobey again?"

"I hope not, Goddess."

"You hope not?"

"Yes, Goddess."

"What does that mean?"

"I do not wish to disobey, Goddess; I did not mean to disobey the first time. But since I made one error I fear the possibility exists that someday I may make another despite my best intentions, Goddess."

You looked at me through a very long silence. You might have been amused or you might have been irritated; I could not tell from your face. "That may be true," you said at last, "but even though I value the truth I am still going to punish you three times: once for your disobedience, once because I don't like the truth you told, and once because I enjoy doing it. Turn around. Face on the ground. Are you ready?"

"Yes, Goddess."

"Ask."

"Please, Goddess, may I have my first punishment?"

You did not wait, you did not warm me up, you gave me no word or sign or warning, you just snapped your wrist down like a gate. I felt the switch and heard the wind it made, then felt the heat, and finally the pain ran along my nerves like a fire through dry leaves.

"One Ma'am," I gasped, "thank you Ma'am. Please, Goddess, may I have my second punishment?"

Again you were neither kind nor cruel, and you did not wait or tease. The switch came down and every step lit up my brain and made my body quiver.

"Two Ma'am, thank you Ma'am. Please, Goddess, may I have my third punishment?"

You brought the cane down softly to my skin and moved it in deft circles on my two fresh stripes while I grew frightened, then impatient, and finally just hungry, my twitching muscles giving me away. You scratched lightly at my welts with your fingernails. "The third punishment I shall hold in abeyance, to deliver any time I see fit. Any time. Any time we should be together – in my house, on a beach, at a party, in the back row of an airplane – any time I believe my special attention is called for I may punish you once more if I want to, and you will ask for it. Do you understand?"

"Yes, Goddess."

"And do you agree?"

"Yes, Goddess."

You bent down and laid the tip of the switch against my lips. "In that case your life is mine," you whispered in my face. "You have the heart of a slave, and I have the heart of a Mistress. I want your soul. I will cut your throat, not deep enough to endanger you, but deep and long enough for you to know I own you beyond recall. I will brand you and pierce you and lock you to my desk by your penis for weeks at a time. You will never be dressed except in clothes I've worn that smell of me, you will never be uncollared, you will never not be freshly marked. You will serve me always, and serve my friends when they come to call, and you will learn to show in front of them the humility I can see is powerful within you, covered as it is today by layers of fear and pride. You will sleep restrained beside me, or on the floor beside my bed at night. Each morning I will re-assert my rights as your owner. You will learn to love the weight of me standing on your flesh. You will learn to love to weep in pain for me. You will please me over and over without your own release until I have a purpose for your orgasm. Look at you, boy: you know I'm speaking to your heart."

I'd grown erect while listening to you, mesmerized by your voice and eyes, mesmerized by what you were saying. You *had* spoken to my heart and oh Goddess! You brought hope and joy to that heart. You took my head from behind with one hand, and brought the other up to caress my cheek. You brought your face close to mine and kissed my eyes. You smiled from deep within you to deep within me and you began to slap my face, gently at first, harder as you worked yourself up, holding my head to keep my neck from snapping, seeing that I hated being slapped, seeing that I loved to give you any gift you wanted. You shook in your own orgasms, and when you were through you took the leash from the collar at my neck and clipped it to the collar at my balls.

You pushed me onto my back and stood over me. I felt your heat descend. I saw you, I smelled you, I let my mouth fall open as you brushed against me. I tasted you, and suddenly, with a flood of blood, my cock grew so hard it ached.

Up and down my face you rubbed yourself, marking me as an animal marks her territory. You pushed yourself onto my forehead, my chin, my nose, my cheeks, my eyes, you wiped yourself in my hair, pressed yourself on my chest, and slid down my body leaving your scent everywhere, returning at last to sit astride my mouth again. "Now, use your tongue. Very slowly. Very soft. Long strokes. To the right. Up. Up. Yes. Yes. Yes."

I lost myself in pleasing you, my senses utterly submerged in you. Now and then I rolled my hips to still the numbness that kept creeping into my hands, now and then I worked a cramp from the muscles of my tongue and jaw, now and then you pulled the leash, reminding me that I belonged to you as I made myself your vehicle and drank you in as you rode me through the afternoon.

If I had had a sense of time before I lost it in the music of your sounds; if I'd had a sense of place I lost it in the pressure of your hips and thighs; if I'd had a sense of me I lost it in my passionate desire to give myself away. I held my mouth in place for you as you came and came in long, drawn-out waves. In the tensions and releases of your climaxes your breath came hard, and with it you laughed and laughed. You braced your feet against my hips, your breasts teased my face, and you stilled slowly down, settling yourself softly in my mouth again.

I wanted to kiss and caress and make love to every part of you. I thought I must be permanently erect. I was close to orgasm myself but knew I was not allowed, so I dropped down and became the sensation, became an extension of my Mistress, my owner, my Goddess, you. I rested my head against your thigh. Peaceful as though your orgasms had been my own, at last I fell into the space you were and vanished.

The sun was setting for the second time. You led me back inside. You took your goblet from the dresser in the bedroom and walked me to the living room where you reclined on the sofa as you had the night before. Your friend leaned back in the chair I'd assumed last night. She found my clothes beneath it and at a nod from you she slowly tore them all apart: pants, shirt, jacket, shorts, socks. She couldn't rend the shoes, but with hardly a glance in my direction she tossed them with the tatters I once had worn onto the ashes in the fireplace, which were grey and cold and fluttered in the breeze the torn cloth made.

You pointed to the hearth and to the brandy glasses we had shared in what seemed to me another life. "I want the fireplace brushed clean," you said, "and the rags and ashes bagged together and put out with the garbage in the garage. I also want you to wash the glasses the next time I send you out of the room."

In one part of my mind I was stunned to see my clothes destroyed, and I thought about the wallet in what had been my hip pants pocket with the money that was mine and the cards that told me who I was. I thought about the keys to what had been my car and what had been my home. I remembered people and places from the life I'd lived before this moment, or the moment before dawn when you first said *down*. I knew I was no longer free, and wondered if I would ever again be free to leave or disobey or disagree with anything you said. But in another part of my mind I also knew that none of my recollections mattered any more. As I stared into your eyes which had gone flat black, I felt I had become an object subject to your mercy or your whims, and I was thrilled.

"Yes, Goddess," I whispered for the form.

You took me by the hair and pulled me forward, then bent me back on my elbows so the front of my body was completely open from my throat down to my parted knees. You left me exposed while you got up off the couch and took the crystal pendant from your neck. You knelt beside me and stared into my eyes, and brought the pendant's point to rest at the base of my penis.

"You are my slave now, is that so?" you asked.

"Yes, Goddess," I replied in terror.

"Is there anything I don't have the right to do to you?"

"No, Goddess."

"Then you'll be happy I'm so kind." You smiled. "At least for now."

You brought the pendant to my breast and drew a sign on me with its icy point. From the corners of my eyes I could see the lines of the sign quickly fill with blood, although I felt no pain. Your eyes glittered like the pendant. You squeezed my cuts and made the blood run freely to your hand, then slapped me and smeared my face with red.

"I hereby claim you, before a woman witness. You will never be free again." You kissed the pendant and held it out for me to kiss, then put it on again. My blood slithered down its length in streaks between your breasts.

You pulled at my legs as if I were an animal, examining my bruised, raw knees. "I don't think you should crawl or kneel much more today," you said. "Soon it will be time for you to prepare dinner. My friend is staying so you will set two places. I will feed you afterwards in some – special – way. But for now you may kiss my feet while I visit with my friend. You are not to *stop* kissing them until I tell you to. Do you understand?"

"Yes, Goddess."

I settled myself on the floor in front of you as comfortably as I could, and for the next long period of time, while you and your friend visited, I made love to your feet with my hands and mouth, kissing, caressing, licking, petting, sucking, till someplace deep inside my soul I had a kind of cosmic orgasm. I didn't come, by which I mean my cock didn't shoot – I didn't have permission to do that in any case – but at another level of my being I found that as I worshipped at the feet of this Goddess in your human form I was also worshipping all the Goddesses, right up to the Great Goddess who creates all life and love and happiness of every kind, and all terror too: She who takes life and love and happiness away; She who is the Mother of the childish, warring gods we human males pretend we're like; She whose power and grandeur reign over all of us like the sky that is Her skirt and the stars that are the jewels She scatters through our mortal heavens so that we may know that She is always there to love and comfort us if only we are willing to come to Her and ask, and say as we may say to Her through all the Godesses on Earth – through our mothers and sisters and wives and girlfriends and colleagues at the office and on the job, through the ticket takers at the movie houses and the waitresses who bring us coffee and the customers we serve in our stores and the women we leave starving on our streets in wounded countries and dying of neglect around the world – and say as we may say to Her through all the Goddesses on Earth, "I love you. I adore you. Thank you for letting me worship at your feet."

An earlier version of this story appeared in Attitude, Issue #6.

Terror, Trance and Transformation[*]

John Dabell

This thing of darkness I acknowledge mine. – William Shakespeare

The fears start to multiply. From a place, shadowy and forbidden, the monstrous shapes usher forth with increasing ferocity. Each fear writhes past my captive mind, settling quickly in a different part of my body. Traveling the crossroads of nerve and blood, they find home in bone and joint, muscle and organ. From their unclaimed past, a lexicon of terrors blossoms forth in the paradise of my soul.

Oh, Threefold Shade, Silent Watcher of the Crossroads,
You who hold the keys to the huge and thoughtful night,
You who hold the keys to the cradle and the grave,
Friend and Fiend of Time, we invoke you.

Hekate, we draw you up from the earth!
Hekate, we draw you forth from the seas!
Hekate, we draw you down from the sky![1]

My body has become a complex landscape of biochemical interactions, of endorphins and adrenaline compounds dialoguing with the mind and

---

[*] I first used the title "Terror, Trance and Transformation" for a workshop created by Joi Wolfwomyn and myself, on the therapeutic use of fear, for PantheaCon 1995. The title continues to be used to describe Joi's continued explorations of the subject.

soul. The scent of my body has changed and, with a mysterious power, all my senses explode. The corners of the room and all secrets of the night are mine to scrutinize in painful detail. I am the raw product of that mix of instinctual alarm and jarring anxiety we call fear.

Mine is the tenth and last body-piercing to be performed tonight. The tension climbs the walls of the room with each new person's ordeal. As the last initiate before me cries out in pain, I search desperately for a way out of the house. Only the numbing prospect of humiliation keeps my two legs from bolting out the door. My initial anxiety of strangers and strange settings has now been replaced by a more visceral fear of needles, blood, and pain.

The beat of my heart has long ceased to be confined to a chest cavity. Its throb extends to the tips of my fingers and toes; my head pounds so loudly, I strain to hear the voice of the High Priest over the waves of dissolution that crash inside my skull.

Oh, Terrible Tomb-frequenter, mystery-raving with souls of the dead,
You, Sacred Shadow of our Thirteenth Hour,
You, still the only One; You, still this Moment,
Divine Impermanence, come dance the Black Void.

Hekate, we draw you up from the earth!
Hekate, we draw you forth from the seas!
Hekate, we draw you down from the sky!

Now I'm lying face up on the central altar, a large, padded, black leather massage table. Two friends position themselves at each side of me and hold my outstretched arms down tight. Another two have positioned themselves at my head and feet and the one at my head covers my face with the ritual shawl. Two new fears, of the dark and being held down, take root in the depths of my imagination. A lost memory, buried since childhood, surfaces and for a moment my kid brother has me trapped in the closet, a cruel menagerie of stuffed creatures pinning me to the closet floor. The High Priest's voice fades in and out. Somehow, his disembodied words get through and I remember to breathe again.

Oh, Delightful Torment, Mauve-hearted Rose, Thorn of my Desire,
You are the knife and the wound, the slap and the cheek,
You are the wheel and the broken limb, hangman and victim both,
Night's Great Vampire at our veins, come feast on our blood.

Hekate, we draw you up from the earth!
Hekate, we draw you forth from the seas!
Hekate, we draw you down from the sky!

I just have time to exhale when searing pain, the color of midnight, slices through my chest. The two hollow needles have been driven through my pink nipples. My consciousness shoots out of the top of my head and oblivion begets a personality. Oblivion begets a particular smell, a particular taste. I know You! Something distinct and recognizable pushes me aside and enters through the hole in the top of my head. I see my body in the center of the room surrounded by attentive friends. They watch as She takes control, a force embodied once again. I watch the process, fascinated by my helplessness. The convulsions make my body look like a human puppet with a finger in the cosmic light-socket. My previous ideas of "pleasure" and "pain" have become two tiny ants squashed beneath the devastating weight of Ecstasy. My lexicon of terrors is put to rest.

"Who sleeps well?" writes Yi-Fu Tuan. "Those who can afford to be unafraid."[2] Fears haunt our childhood, our adolescence, and later maturity. Triggered by both physical and psycho-spiritual situations, fear conditions us, limits us. Its ever-fluid landscape subjects us to a constant ebb and flow of anxiety as new subjects for alarm emerge and disappear from the daily history. Fear necessitates that we create boundaries to keep our lives "safe." It helps to shape our understanding of "reality."

But how we experience the devastation of flood or drought, disease or deformity, or even the sight of a corpse torn apart by war depends on the historical context. Our position relative to history makes our reaction to fear obviously unique from that of any other age. As we map and re-map our known world, our fears shift and modify themselves. The faces of many of our fears disappear, others just become more manageable.

Sometimes the voices of our anxieties speak more softly, other times they will speak no more. When the destructive temperament of a hurricane is statistically analyzed and the meteorological science of "prediction" saves the lives and property of thousands with advanced notice, the "wrath of the Gods" becomes just a whim of nature.

But, unfortunately, many of our fears persist. The fear of death is, perhaps, the most pernicious, haunting us over the course of our lives. We go to great lengths to circumvent that final moment. We take out all manner of "insurance," from the deals we make with "God" to the deals we make with life-insurance brokers. The fear of dying maps out our lives in subtle ways too. We change our diet and wear our seat-belts. We fetishize all manner of things in our lives with hopes of delaying the inevitable. The simple ritual, for instance, of the "one-a-day" vitamin holds a near-mystical power, able to vanquish all manner of "ills" with a single pill. Our pursuit of health is, in part, the constructive management of our fears around dying.

My maternal grandmother died as the direct result of a physician's misdiagnosis, when I was eight. Her death was my first encounter with the tenuous quality of life. I was barely able to comprehend the magnitude of our parting, let alone understand how such an event could have been brought about by someone my grandmother had entrusted with her well-being. The impressions her accidental death left followed me from childhood into adulthood. While many of the impressions were far from comfortable, two direct and positive results of the event were a career in holistic healing and working with the elderly.

But my grandmother's death provoked another result. My personal relationship to the mystical was born out of my need to put death and the process of dying into a larger, more holistic framework. I searched for dynamic, alternative models for traversing the landscape of fear that a Euro-colonialist, hetero-patriarchal culture had created around me. The resurgence of European pre-Christian spiritual traditions, popularized by many feminists and the Neo-Pagan communities, helped me to find my way to the feet of Hekate, the Great Dark Mother, "the Beginning and the End, and... Mistress of All."[3]

Hekate played a central role in the pantheistic religions of Eastern Europe and Asia Minor. Her worship is part of a much larger landscape of Goddess worship in Asia Minor, the Aegean and Balkan areas that dates back 8000 to 9000 years. The archetypal "Bitch Goddess," Hekate is perhaps best known as "Queen of the Witches," wandering crossroads with Her hordes of demon hounds, by the dark of the new moon. Shakespeare casts Her opposite Macbeth in his famous play. We envision Her as an ancient crone who is called upon to aid witches in nefarious spell casting or as the ancient guardian to the underworld of our collective unconscious. She fuses with the image of Holda, a Teutonic "underworld" deity, and we see Her riding Her broom across Halloween's night sky. She survives as La Befanna in Italy, bringing toys to good children and candy "coal" to bad ones on January sixth. Young or old, we approach Her with great respect, in part out of fear of Her dread reputation.

Despite Her "survival" in our popular imagination, the cultural fears of dominant women and autonomous sexuality mix with fears of an untamed nature, the dark night, aging and death, allowing us to experience only a very limited part of Hekate. Arguably one of the most dynamic and functional expressions of the "Bitch Goddess" archetype in the ancient Mediterranean world, Hekate has been reduced to an almost comic-book caricature of Her former glory. Worshipped since at least the eighth century B.C.E., Her worship spans many countries and cultures, and She runs an associative gamut from chthonic to celestial, terrifying to beneficent. Her primary priesthood were the *demosioi* (also known as the *semnotatoi*), a gender-variant and homoerotically inclined cast of eunuchs, similar to the *galli*, the eunuch priests of Cybele. The tradition of gender variance and ritual homoerotic behavior dates as far back as 3000 B.C.E. in Phrygia, the home of Hekate worship.[5]

In *The Golden Ass*, written in the second century C.E. by Apuleius, the hero Lucius prays to the moon. He calls Her Regina Caeli, "Queen of

Heaven," a title which would later be given to the Virgin Mary. When Lucius falls asleep, the Goddess appears to him, revealing Her true power.

> I am the mother of the nature of things, the mistress of all the elements, the original progeny of the ages, the supreme divinity, queen of the departed souls, chief of the deities of heaven, the manifestation in one of all the gods and goddesses. By my commands, I regulate the bright vault of heaven, the health-giving sea breezes, the bereaved silence of the dead.

The Queen of Heaven goes on to proclaim what will become a major building block of Jungian psychology, the writings of Joseph Campbell and the Neo-Pagan revival of the 20th century:

> The whole world venerates my single name in many forms, with varied ritual, with a name linked to many others. And so the Phrygians, the first born of all humans, call me Mother of the Gods at Pessinus; native Athenians call me Cecropean Minerva; the sea-tossed Cyprians, Paphian Venus; the Cretan archers, Diana Dictynna; the tri-lingual Sicilians, Stygian Proserpine; the Eleusinians, the most ancient goddess Ceres. Some call me Juno, others Bellona. Here I am Hekate...

While Apuleius's narrative reads like a piece of Roman propaganda with its idea of an "officially sanctioned" deity unifying the various religions of conquered people, the passage also demonstrates the scope of a bitch goddess archetype and Hekate's influence on the popular mind as Her worship spread from Phrygia throughout the classical world.

In the Ancient and Classical world, artists, priests, philosophers, and magicians portrayed Hekate as exercising dominion over everything from the earth to the heavens, as associated with both the moon and the sun, and as ensouling the cosmos and giving birth to the universe. She was associated with hunting and farming, poisoning and healing, death and the birth process. She aided the warrior and the athlete, kings and fishermen; She was Hekate, the Great Dark Mother, "the Beginning and the End, and... Mistress of All."

But, beneath the veil of Hekate's infinite power lies a more significant subtlety. In Hesiod's seventh-century B.C.E. cosmological poem "Theogony" (one of the earliest written records of Hekate in Greek mythology), Zeus bestows a share of the earth and the seas on Hekate, "whom Zeus honored above all," and commands that She be honored in the starry heavens by the deathless gods. Zeus's unequaled generosity is a recognition of Hekate's implicit autonomy. Her power of self-governance, power independent of lineage or procreative obligation, commands respect from the greatest of the Olympians. It is this implicit autonomy that is the true source of the Bitch's archetypal power. Self-assured and self-possessed, Hekate represents the very essence of control. Mistress of Fate, She holds the keys to the universe.

In the *Orphic Hymns*, She is called the "Key-Holding Queen of the Entire Cosmos." The title key-holder is frequently applied to Her, as well as a number of other Greek Gods. From archaic times the word was used metaphorically to express that someone was master or mistress of whatever the key in question unlocked. The key-holder controls the access between the realms. The keys held by Hekate opened the gates of Hades and in the Greek Magical Papyri the keys are said to open the "bars of Cerberus," the three-headed dog that guards the realm of the dead, so that the living cannot enter and the dead cannot leave.[8]

As the key-holding mistress, Hekate holds the power to mediate between worlds. At the threshold between the world of the living and the world of the dead, She stands as guard and guide. Fears necessitate boundaries, a marker and barrier to the "unknown," a threshold beyond which we risk life and limb traversing. Liminal points delineate the differences between two areas or aspects, providing a link to and from these areas, connecting them and mediating between them. Here is the border point between the intelligible world and the sensible world, a threshold not quite belonging to the upper world, not quite belonging to the underworld. At the outermost edge of our safe little world, Hekate silently awaits us, guarding secret wisdom, ready to guide us should we choose to leave the safety of what we've grown to know all too well.

In the same way that Hekate, the "Key-Holding Queen," controlled access between the realms and mediated between the worlds, so did the *demosioi*. In Lagina, Hekate's eunuch priesthood served as ritual intercessors at the annual festival "of the Key," along with choirs of flower-garlanded boys singing hymns of praise. The *demosioi*, a name suggesting "belonging to a tribe," underwent ritual castration and stepped outside the limits of male (by societal definition) and female. Ritually renouncing the societal power derived from either extreme they consciously stepped outside the limits of gender to embrace the power of the liminal state. At the threshold between the world of men and the world of women, they stood as guides and mediators of their culture, casting horoscopes, performing spells, and maintaining Hekate's sacred sites.[10] They served as mediators between the world of humans and those of the Gods, between the living and the dead. They unified the worlds and reveled in the limbo of the in-between, the mystical realm that eludes control or categorization.

Great attention was paid to the threshold in the ancient world. Caves, doors to homes, temples, palaces, and cities were the domain of Hekate. In one respect the threshold represents beginnings, the point at which one departs from one place to enter another. This journey can be physical and symbolic. In a ritual that survives to this day, the Roman bridegroom carried his bride over the threshold. If the transition from single to married life was to be completed successfully, it must be done auspiciously and cautiously, with the help of the Gods. This custom insured that the couple's passage into life together was not marred by a stumbling step.[11]

Because, by its nature, the threshold was distinct from its surroundings, neither belonging to the inside nor outside of the house, violations of this boundary and the implied disregard for limits were seen as bringing disaster. The liminality of thresholds, gates, crossroads and frontiers was viewed as a limbo of possible chaos, with the limen eluding control and categorization. It belonged to no one and was not associated with either extremity divided. It is because of these associations that crossroads became the realm for daemons[12] and spirits of the dead. On a more literal level, it also became associated with prostitutes, thieves, and other personae dispelled from society.[13]

Hekate, as associated with crossroads, had the adjective Edonia regularly applied to Her. It is a term that specifically refers to the place where three points meet. Many crossroads for the Greeks and the Romans were marked by shrines, statues, and sacred stones. The Greeks used special boundary stones to establish the limits of sacred precincts, to delineate the property of the Gods from those of the people. Small altars were set up by the Romans on small boundaries of untilled land where four farm plots met. These altars were to protect the rights of all four landholders.

A multitude of offerings was laid at crossroads at the full moon[14], as well as, most importantly, the new moon to supplicate and placate Hekate. Garlic, honey, eggs, sprat, mullet, cakes and breads, black lambs, dogs, and oxen were all part of the sacrifice laid out as part of the Hekate "Suppers." These elaborate rituals were used as a means to avert the *enthumion*, the easily roused wrath of Hekate and Her daemons. The suppers to Hekate were a form of expiation, a ritual prescription for daily transgressions. The rituals provided the necessary purification for safe passage through one's daily world. Taking offerings to the crossroads at the new moon granted safe passage not only through the physical world (i.e., crossroads) but also, on a symbolic level, between one state of consciousness and another.

By the 2nd century C.E., popularized through the writings of the *Chaldean Oracles*, chthonic Hekate's associations with liminality became fused together with Hellenistic views of the moon and the Platonic concept of a Cosmic Soul. Hekate shifted from being a primarily chthonic deity and developed a strong celestial overtone that had implications for Her worship by the *demosioi* and the general populace. She was placed in a complex cosmological view of the heavens, with the moon becoming the mediating point for passage of Hekate's daemons to and from the heavens, traveling between the earthly and celestial realms.

A collection of ritual oracles, the *Chaldean Oracles* were the written words of Julian "the theurgist," written down by his father, Julian "the Chaldean," while the former spoke for the Gods in trance. The Oracles are part of a rich age in the writings of religious texts of all kinds. The Oracles, fragmented though they are, are the only esoteric religious teachings to have survived on a Goddess from the ancient Greco-Roman world. The *Chaldean Oracles* enjoyed a high status during the Renaissance where, mistakenly attributed to Zoroaster, they formed part of a select group of magical works including the Hermetica, the *Orphic Hymns* and other works attributed to "ancient theologians."[15]

Unfortunately, with the rise in popularity of Hekate and Her evolution to "Mistress of All," Her worship became the precept of theurgist and magicians, who called on Her to do their bidding, like a servant, and set Her into an engendered, hierarchical system requiring elaborate magical operations and incantations to access Her power. Ecstatic worship by the demosioi was displaced by the ceremonial obligations of theurgists and the elaborate spells of magicians.

With the triumph of Christianity over paganism, Hekate's eunuch priesthood, dancing between the worlds, was slowly driven from Her limen and into extinction by progressive waves of Christian influence, reacting in horror to their gender-variant and homoerotic celebration of the ancient Goddess. Fear of the demosioi led to the destruction of their sacred temples and their ecstatic celebrations. Little remains of the power they brought through from their journeys into the forbidden realms beyond the safety of the known. We are left with few clues to their rituals or what they may have seen staring into the eyes of the triple-headed Hekate, as they stood at the crossroads by the dark of the moon, listening to the hidden sounds of the night. What could we have learned from them about navigating our landscapes of fear?

As a priest of Hekate, I walk to the edge of my safe known and wait for Her call. I offer Her honey and pomegranates and wait for Her invitation. Reciting words from Her glorious past, I call Her to me.

For from you are All things, and in you, Eternal One, do All things end.... I offer you this incense... Arrow-shooter, Heavenly One, Goddess of Harbors, Mountain-roamer, Goddess of Crossroads, Nocturnal One of the Underworld, Shadowy One of Hades, Still One who frightens, having feast among the graves. You are Night, Darkness and broad Chaos, For you are Necessity hard to escape, You are Fate, you are Erinys and the Torture, You are the Murderess and Justice, You hold Cerberus in chains, You are steely-blue with serpent-scales, O serpent-haired and Serpent-girdled One, Blood-drinker, Death-bringer who breeds corruption, Feaster on hearts, Flesh-eater who devours those who died before their time, Grave-resounder, Driver to the Wanderings of Madness, Come to my sacrifices....

"Who sleep well?" echoes through the dark.

"Those who can afford to be unafraid," I offer back to Her.

"Who sleep well?"

"Those who dare to see."

She smiles and hands me back a small piece of myself.

1. *Ritual invocation to Hekate adapted from the Orphic Hymns, the Greek Mgical Papyri, the works of Charles Baudelaire, and Tom Johnson.*

2. *Tuan, Yi-Fu*, Landscapes of Fear, *University of Minnesota Press, 1979, p. 4.*

3. *Deitter-Betz, Hans Ed.*, Greek Magical Papyri In Translation, *University of Chicago, 1992 (PGM IV 2785 2870).*

4. *Joseph Campbell, in* The Masks of God, *Vol I-IV, Arkana, New York 1964, cites worship of an archetypal "Great Goddess" in Asia Minor dating back at least 8,000 years. Marija Gimbutas, in The Goddesses and Gods of FOld Europe, University of California Press, Berkeley and Los Angeles, 1982, cites worship in the Aegean and Balkan area to be around 9,000 years old.*

5. *Conner, Randy P.*, Blossom of Bone, *Harper, San Francisco 1993, page 88.*

6. *Lowe, J.E., Magic and Greek and Latin Literature, Oxford 1929, pages 11-15.*

7. *Farnell, I.R., The Cults of the Greek States, Oxford 1896, p. 18. As Hekate's worship spread from Asia Minor into popular Greek and, later, into Roman culture, writers searched for a way to incorporate the non-Greek, older Hekate into their mythology, with its emphasis on lineage. Baccylides called Her the child of Night, Apollodorus said Her mother and father were Asteria and Jove. Lycophron makes Her the daughter of Perses and Hesiod writes, "Phoebe bare Asteria whom Perses led to his house to be called his wife, and she bore Hekate, whoom Zeus honored above all." In the Orphic Hymns, we find that Ceres is called the motehr of FHekate. There was no fixed or accpted genealogy for Hekate. By the second century C.E., She was simply addressed as "the Begining and the End," with emphasis being placed on Her cosmological function.*

8. *Johnston, Sarah Iles,* Hekate Soteira, *Scholars Press, Atlanta, 1990, pps. 40-41.*

9. *Farnell, L.R., op. cit., p. 22.*

10. *Conner, Randy P., op. cit., pps. 83-131.*

11. *Johnston, Sarah Iles, op. cit., p. 25.*

12. *Daemons, writes Johnston (ibid., p. 34), are from their earliest portrayals inphilosophical and mystical writings creatures of mediation or creatures in transition. With Xenocrates, the definition of daemons finds its fullest expression as a class between the Gods and humans. The status of daemons as creatures between the realms parallels the status of eunuchs as beings between the world of men and women, Gods and humans.*

13. *Johnston, Sarah Iles, ibid., p. 26.*

14. *Smith, K.F., "Hekate's Suppers," in the* Encyclopedia of Religion and Ethics, *ed. James Hastings, Edinburgh 1937, Vol. II, pps. 57-63.*

15. *ed. Ronan, Stephen,* The Goddess Hekate, *Chthonios Books, Hastings 1992, pps. 80-81.*

16. *ed. Deitter-Betz, Hans, op. cit. PGM IV 2785 2870.*

Firewheel

Jezebel Strong

Invocation

"Great Spirit, Grant us the serenity to accept the things we cannot change, the courage to change the things we can, and the wisdom to know the difference."

I take her open face into both of my hands and lovingly pour myself into her eyes.

"My sweet boy, tonight I will take you on the journey of the tenth card of the tarot – The Wheel of Fortune. Once I let go of your face you are not to look me in the eyes, you are never to turn your back on me unless told to do so, and you are not to speak unless it is to ask to speak. I do not want you to be uncomfortable so you must communicate any of your physical or emotional needs to me immediately. For example, if your back hurts in a particular position, ask to speak and when I reply, address me formally and with a simple statement such as, 'Mistress, my back hurts on the left in this position'. We create this form and these boundaries in order to journey safely and deeply into and out of ourselves and each other."

After my words of beginning I pull her by the nape of her neck firmly and steadily to her knees. My boy is a tall and elegant butch and a rush always fills my medium frame when she lets me overpower her so willingly.

This initial rush moistens my thighs and I can sense that tonight's venture into the realm of Sex Magic will carry us deep into Persephone's cave of bat wings and pomegranates. I will have my boy eat ten seeds of the bittersweet fruit.

The Climb and Descent

Once my boy is on her knees and I am wet I leave her alone in the very small bedroom with black and cranberry candles burning. I take this time to consider my tools carefully. When I return I lay them out with precision. I am dressed in black lace, heels, and dark scarlet lipstick. My long hair is caught up in two wispy braids and a homemade crown of silver and purple ribbons adorns my head. My earrings are symbols of Goddess power – moons and stars. All of this is important for me as I open to the climb into my power, just as the simple nakedness of my boy helps her descend. When I have determined that she is deserving I will place her leather collar on her neck – until then I let only the candlelight and my gloved hands cover her.

I turn on the tape I have prepared – ten versions of the Grateful Dead's "The Wheel." My boy grins and lifts her eyes as far as my cheeks. She feels how deeply I know her musician self to have chosen thus. I allow her this moment of recognition and stand assured in her gaze.

As the music begins to rise in rhythm I pull my boy onto the bed – her ass against the soft quilt, arms and legs spread to the four corners. A full silence begins to fill my mind. I know I am reaching the top of my inner ascent when I begin to hear quiet. I take each of her wrists and buckle her in securely, hook her to the chains attached to the upper corner posts. I tell her to remain completely still and if she is able to do so I will kindly restrain her legs. As she settles into her self-imposed stillness, I pick out my favorite and her least favorite toy. Sometimes this boy needs a slow fall, but on this night of fierce magic I want her to crash down. The rod is very very thin and accurate. The pain it creates in my hand is focused. I pick a meaty place on her long left thigh and bring the rod down with some force. My boy winces but does not move. I take the snap of pain to her right thigh and she remains still. Now that she is doing exactly what I want I feel enticed to challenge her and a storm of rod blows falls on her. Through it all she grimaces, sighs in delight, moans, and remains still. It is time to reward her with the completion of four point bondage. My Apache ancestors come into the room and tell a story about the importance of the directions. My boy listens to this wisdom with rapt attention – totally aware that our souls have reached the point of openness.

The Heart

Once the directions have been acknowledged it is time to burn sage to be certain that the space we are entering is purified. My boy breathes the sweet smoke in and arches her body into the warmth of the small flame. Her longing is written on her in sweat. Her armpits shine. Her open thighs release her scent into the room. The feast of smells plays with the liquid sound of Garcia's guitar. I am soaring. I feel wings all around me. I give my boy her collar and she lets another layer fall. Putting the sage aside I take up a red candle and create a wheel of wax on my boy's belly. She dances into each drip of the hot wax and her patterned movement invites us both into a heartbeat rhythm. I drip the wax in time with the drums. The wax gets thick and her belly becomes the visual center of our ritual. I add a feathered clothespin to the display, drop some ice in the center and talk to her of the significance of the elements – air, fire, water and earth. Her hunger for my words is matched by her desire for sensation.

I pick up my favorite deep red and black whip and work steadily on her already welt-covered thighs. My boy is pulling hard against her restraints and dancing with the small freedom of movement she has been given. We both receive the significant sounds of the Dead now and repetition has worked us into timelessness. I begin chanting the words, "you are a Jew. I am a Jew," over and over. "We move with Shekinah. We dance with the Tree of Life." She hears me but doesn't seem to hear the words as anything other than sound, which is exactly what I want – meaning without effort. I let my Jewish soul speak to her. With each fall of the whip another word of life comes from the inside of me, "Source," "Power," "Prayer," "Perseverance," "Peace," "Awareness." I end – as the music gentles – with, "As a Jew you are invited to argue with Spirit." My boy growls and flashes her teeth at me. We have reached the center of her submission/masochism and my dominance/sadism. I feed her the ten bittersweet seeds of the pomegranate.

The Lesson

Now I call up the image of the tenth card of the tarot for her and remind her of Ezekiel's vision of the beasts on the firewheel. I ask her to tell me of these beasts. She has let go of most of the connections between speech and thought. Slowly, she is able to name the bull, human and lion, but she can not find the word for eagle. She calls it a "chicken-headed thing," and we burst into peals and gales of laughter. We cannot stop laughing. We cry and laugh and laugh and cry. I then take the scalpel and hold it up so that the edge is playing with candlelight. She is instantly still. My boy's breathing slows. I take the blade and enter her chest to re-mark her on a cutting that we have returned to many times. As her skin separates she smiles. The smell of her blood consumes us both and with precision and grace I cut and she breathes. Tears trickle from the sides of her eyes and she is smiling. "This is your lesson, my boy," I say in a low voice and then I repeat to her the lyrics of "The Wheel" by Robert Hunter:

> The Wheel is turning
> and you can't slow it down
> You can't let go
> and you can't hold on
> You can't go back
> and you can't stand still
> If the thunder don't get you
> then the lightning will....

"I am your thunder and your lightning, my boy."

The Connection

I rub alcohol on her cutting to add a quick burn to the mark and then I free her arms. My boy speaks on her own for the first time, "Mistress, may I speak?"

"Yes, my boy."

"Mistress, may I embrace you and hold you to me?"

The Prayer of Completion

"Great Spirit, grant us the serenity to accept the things we cannot change, the courage to change the things we can, and the wisdom to know the difference."

Worshipping

Sossity Oessa Chiricuzio

Why are you here with me now, in this place full and roiling with the smoke of musk and cabalistic desire? It is a magic I will weave of the self strands you offer – pysche, sex and old old pain. It was lived in this flesh your flesh and so there the release
You offer up your back to me arms wide enough to fly
ragged breaths
rooted deep in your throat
my presence behind you
& this leather freight train
are all that you know of gravity
It is this sacred animal lore – the knowledge of pain and the sweetest twisting of nerves – you seek in my hands, in my motherwit. I will not lull you or leave you to drift in amorphous pleasure. I want your focus hard, I want you to throb with the melting wisdom of your self as the tears wash through your crevassed soul and we sweat together
endorphins
heat shuddering across skin gone electric thin
I will see you dance a wild howling
as the shadows peel away from your incandescent flesh
Your blood knows me – Beast Goddess – as I bite with your own hunger. I am come to open you up to the wild night air, the cold steel edge of the moon, the heat of my rough honeyed tongue. My energy into your body into my body into your energy

this violet loop is the blessing

the feeding

the ritual

My love – you have only to ask for my blue fire, the depths of my body, my queer queer knowledge of your ancient girlchild wounds... and I will climb under your bones and touch you behind your heart.

Contributors' Notes

Once described as "Oscar Wilde in a corset," **Christina Abernathy** has made it her life's work to instruct submissives in the finer points of service. When she isn't busy doling out proper sets of six, Miss Abernathy enjoys baroque chamber music, tea in her rose garden, and edifying reading.

Lady Bachu writes from a ridge-top in the sensuous Sonoma wine region of Northern California. A lesbian Priestess/poet, she is a co-founder of the MoonWyse coven. Her current projects include a collection of short stories and poetry called *In the Temple of the Sacred Whore*.

Now that she is over 40, **Pat Califia** feels free to write about topics that are even more shocking than sadomasochism – for example, goddess worship. Among other things, she is the author of two sex manuals, *Sapphistry* and *Sensuous Magic*, two short story collections, *Macho Sluts* and *Melting Point*, one novel, *Doc and Fluff*, a collection of essays, *Public Sex*, a poetry collection, *Diesel Fuel*, and has edited *Doing It For Daddy*, *The Second Coming* (with Robin Sweeney) and *Between Our Lips*, a collection of erotic lesbian poetry. In the works is a second novel, *The Code*, and *The Crook and the Flail: Spirituality and Radical Sex*, forthcoming from Masquerade Books.

Drew Campbell is a female-to-male transsexual writer/editor and spiritual seeker. Writing as his femme alter ego, Christina Abernathy, Drew is the author of *Miss Abernathy's Concise Slave Training Manual* (San Francisco: Greenery Press, 1996). He lives with his beloved and their three cats in San Francisco.

Sossity Oessa Chiricuzio writes, "I am a working class/poor, hippy-raised. freak, Sicilian/white trash, femme queer. I write about those things that grip my gut: sex, gender, work, flesh, power, emotion, ritual, connection, spirituality. My other 'writer's gold star' at this printing is a short story in the anthology *The Second Coming:* 'and I called her boy...' Contact from writers/queers invited: catwench@nakedpc.com."

John Dabell is a traditional herbalist who specializes in the shamanic uses of entheogenic plants, especially the Nightshade family. He teaches classes in shamanism and is currently researching the role of eunuchs in the worship of Hekate. His writings have appeared in *RFD* and *Widdershins*.

Dossie Easton's poetry has appeared under the pen name "Scarlet Woman" in various anthologies, including *Coming to Power* and *The Second Coming*. She is co-author of three books, *The Bottoming Book, or How To Get Terrible Things Done To You By Wonderful People; The Topping Book, or Getting Good At Being Bad;* and *The Ethical Slut: A Guide to Infinite Sexual Possibilities*. Dossie is a therapist in private practice in San Francisco, and she lives in the mountains of Marin, where she declaims poetry to the crows and hosts seriously outrageous pajama parties.

Nicola Ginzler's work appears in *The Second Coming* (Alyson Publications, 1996) and a number of national and international magazines. She has read and performed her work in San Francisco, L.A., Boston, and New York. Her collection of short fiction and poems, *Claustrophobia & Other Stories*, will appear in 1998.

Joi Wolfwomyn, aka Wolfie, is a pagan priest, hippie-anarchist welfare mother living in Oakland, with dreams of opening a temple/dungeon in Oregon sometime in the next five years. When pressed, she identifies politically as a drag queen leatherdyke separatist. She prefers to call her followers "devotees" rather than "slaves," because they have to be seriously devoted to put up with her, especially during her bouts with fibromyalgia. Currently creating a family with Robin Sweeney and her eleven-year-old daughter, she dreams of a day when polyfidelity and polyamorous are everyday words and the day when her daughter is done with puberty.

Liz Highleyman is a writer and health educator. Her work has appeared in *Bi Any Other Name, The Second Coming,* and *Whores and Other Feminists*.

She is the associate editor of *Bisexual Politics: Theories, Queries and Visions* and is editor of the pansexual SM magazine *Cuir Underground*.

Raven Kaldera has been an astrologer and priest/ess of the Dark Goddess and the Lord of the Dead for a decade and currently runs Cauldron Farm, a pagan ecogarden and temple. Raven has been published in Circlet Press's *Blood Kiss, S/M Futures, Genderflex,* and *Worlds of Women II*.

Jad Keres writes, "I'm a 48-year-old dyke living in Eastern Pennsylvania. Born catholic and born again pagan and finally discovering what it means to be alive. Look out world!"

Catherine A. Liszt is a writer, publisher, mother, switchable top, and pain fetishist living in San Francisco, in an ever-shifting polyamorous household anchored by herself and her partner. She has written or co-authored a total of six books under this name and her other pseudonym "Lady Green."

Laurie LoveKraft, also known as Laurie K.Y., holds a Master's in Cultural Anthropology and is a writer, performer, and ritualist. A veteran of the San Francisco sex industry, Laurie is also a ten-year magickal practitioner. Her work has appeared in *Green Egg, Widdershins,* and *Perceptions Magazine*, and she recently released her first book of poetry entitled *Scarlet Letters, Black & Blue*.

Heather MacAllister is "female (born and living as), 28, white, fat, femme, fatale, mixed-class background, currently able-bodied, is working towards the end of oppression in the sexiest and most entertaining way she can find." Look for her in *Fat Girl* magazine. She is called Mistress (Lucretia Morgan) by a fortunate few.

MATAKLAR is a play persona of Ketti Neil, an artist and art theorist living in Philadelphia. "The Sacred Prostitute and the Three Kings" evolved out of a real life search for temple slaves and was first presented as a performance reading at a queer "women's brothel night" in 1994.

John McClimans, long-time Spiral member and priest, died at his home on the night of November 10, 1996, surrounded by family and friends. John's involvement in the pagan community began in Chicago in the 1960s. He was a founding member of the Church of All Worlds. He was also a third degree initiate of a Gardnerian coven, an active member of The Covenant of the Goddess, and a Red Cord initiate in NROOGD, among other affiliations.

Ian Philips is the managing editor for the Damron Company. At the onset of his Saturn return, the Furies ordered him to write more, edit less. He hopes this first public offering will soften their hearts enough to allow him a boyfriend or an agent while he completes the other chapters from their novel, *St. Gawkward of Tulsa*.

Lori Selke lives in San Francisco. Her work has previously appeared in the 'zines *Black Sheets* and *Fat Girl*, and in the anthologies *The Second Coming* (Alyson) and *Genderflex* (Circlet Press), and is forthcoming in the anthology *Leatherwomen III* (Masquerade). She enjoys being lovingly and consensually bossy.

Jezebel Strong (aka "jezi") has a piece in *The Second Coming* entitled "Ball and Chain." She is happy to still be attached! Jezebel longs for more freedom for queers and so she spends the wee hours writing wild words, playing, and praying. "Firewheel" is a "true story."

Robin Sweeney is a writer, editor, and cyberspace content manipulator – how's that for a job description – living in Oakland, California. She is the co-editor, with Pat Califia, of *The Second Coming* (Alyson Publications, 1996) and is working on a novel. She can always be found at robsweeney@aol.com.

Lamar Van Dyke is a visual artist, tattoo artist, writer and thinker who has been living in Seattle for the past 17 years. She is a founding member of Outer Limits, the Seattle Lesbian SM group, and is also a founding member of Powersurge. She has done extensive hands-on research into the realms of SM and is a contributor to *The Second Coming*.

She likes to have fun, take risks, fly high, and push everyone's limits including her own.

James Williams' work has appeared in such magazines as *Advocate Men, Sandmutopia Guardian, Spectator,* and *Black Sheets*, and in numerous anthologies including *Doing It for Daddy* (edited by Pat Califia), *SM Futures* (edited by Cecilia Tan), and *Best American Erotica 1995* (edited by Susie Bright). He lives reclusively in San Francisco.

Maude Wolff is the pseudonym of a Bay Area writer, gardener, and SM practitioner.

Dragon Xcalibur is a butch Top, an androgyne, a ferryman, and a faerie man, who honors the Goddess all ways, and who will sit willingly, joyfully, obediently at Her right hand, when it is She who asks.

Other Books from Greenery Press

The Bottoming Book: Or, How To Get Terrible Things Done To You By Wonderful People
Dossie Easton & Catherine A. Liszt, illustrated by Fish $11.95

Bottom Lines: Poems of Warmth and Impact
H. Andrew Swinburne, illustrated by Donna Barr $9.95

The Compleat Spanker
Lady Green $11.95

The Ethical Slut: A Guide to Infinite Sexual Possibilities
Dossie Easton & Catherine A. Liszt $15.95

A Hand in the Bush: The Fine Art of Vaginal Fisting
Deborah Addington $11.95

KinkyCrafts: 101 Do-It-Yourself S/M Toys
compiled and edited by Lady Green with Jaymes Easton $19.95

Miss Abernathy's Concise Slave Training Manual
Christine Abernathy $11.95

Sex Toy Tricks: More than 125 Ways to Accessorize Good Sex
Jay Wiseman $11.95

The Sexually Dominant Woman: A Workbook for Nervous Beginners
Lady Green $11.95

SM 101: A Realistic Introduction - 2nd Edition
Jay Wiseman $24.95

Supermarket Tricks: More than 125 Ways to Improvise Good Sex
Jay Wiseman $11.95

The Topping Book: Or, Getting Good At Being Bad
Dossie Easton & Catherine A. Liszt, illustrated by Fish $11.95

Tricks: More than 125 Ways to Make Good Sex Better
Jay Wiseman $11.95

Tricks 2: Another 125 Ways to Make Good Sex Better
Jay Wiseman $11.95

Coming in 1998

Juice: Electricity for Pleasure and Pain, by "Uncle Abdul" and Jay Wiseman

Please include $3 for first book and $1 for each additional book with your order
to cover shipping and handling costs. VISA/MC accepted. Order from:

greenery press

3739 Balboa #195, San Francisco, CA 94121
toll-free: 888/944-4434   fax: 415/242-4409   http://www.bigrock.com/~greenery